MEDITATION
SECRETS
FOR WOMEN

MEDITATION SECRETS FOR WOMEN

Discovering Your Passion, Pleasure, and Inner Peace

CAMILLE MAURINE & LORIN ROCHE, Ph.D.

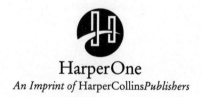

HarperOne
An Imprint of HarperCollinsPublishers

HarperOne

MEDITATION SECRETS FOR WOMEN: *Discovering Your Passion, Pleasure, and Inner Peace.*
Copyright © 2001 by Camille Maurine and Lorin Roche. All rights reserved.
Printed in the United States of America. No part of this book may be used or reproduced
in any manner whatsoever without written permission except in the case of brief quotations
embodied in critical articles and reviews. For information address HarperCollins Publishers,
10 East 53rd Street, New York, NY 10022.

HarperCollins books may be purchased for educational, business, or sales promotional use.
For information please write: Special Markets Department, HarperCollins Publishers,
10 East 53rd Street, New York, NY 10022.

HarperCollins Web site: http://www.harpercollins.com
HarperCollins®, ▇ ®, and HarperOne™ are trademarks of HarperCollins Publishers.

Library of Congress Cataloging-in-Publication Data
Maurine, Camille.
Meditation secrets for women : discovering your passion, pleasure, and inner peace /
Camille Maurine & Lorin Roche.
p.   cm.
Includes bibliographical references.
ISBN 978–0–06–251697–8
1. Meditation 2. Women—Psychology.   I Roche, Lorin.   II Title.
BF637.M4 M7 2000
158.1'2'082—dc21   00-058053

14 15 16 RRD(H) 20 19 18 17 16 15

To all the women of wisdom throughout the ages

❧

To those who have found their voice,
and those who have worked quietly behind the scenes

❧

To the joyous Dakinis who have shared their secrets

Contents

Preface

This book grew out of a lively conversation with my husband Lorin that began when we met in 1983 and continues to this day. We both teach meditation and often discuss the interplay of meditation with love, work, play, creativity, and health. One of our central subjects is how meditation can be integrated into the challenges and joys of modern life.

We both feel immeasurably blessed by the ancient traditions, particularly those of Asia. But the field of meditation has been not just a man's world but a monk's world. For thousands of years monks have been the primary custodians of the knowledge of meditation and the creators of its techniques, so naturally it has been designed to meet their needs. Consequently, most teachings on meditation are still shaped by attitudes that worked in the distant past, in the Far East, for reclusive and celibate males. Far too little is known about what works for women, especially contemporary women. Meditation is slowly being adapted to the West, but the time has come for a new focus, one that specifically addresses women's needs and strengths.

Since the mid-1970s I have been teaching meditation primarily in the context of movement, combining inner awareness with outer expression. Over this time countless women have shared their discoveries as we've explored the depths of female experience. Lorin has been a meditation teacher since 1970. When he coaches people, Lorin likes to find out about their lives—their longings, their loves, their innate wisdom. Rather than impose rigid techniques, he helps them customize their practice to suit their individual nature.

Lorin is always researching what works. One morning right after I'd been meditating he asked, "What do women need to know to thrive in meditation?"

As I answered from the meditative state, he wrote down what I said on five-by-eight cards and spread them out on the rug. Later, as we gazed at the cards, I mused, "You know, these really are secrets. These principles are not what people usually think of as meditation, but they are vitally important for women. Most teachings just do not comprehend the female body and psyche." Lorin then suggested, "Why not write about this so that more women can know?" At first I dismissed the idea because I had my hands full with other creative projects. But then, an alarming number of friends and clients—highly educated and spiritually oriented women—began confiding to me that they were taking antidepressants. Their depression and anxiety seemed to be eloquent expressions of a larger cultural dynamic: the urgent need for women to reclaim their inner ground. I became ever more impassioned and rededicated to these issues, Lorin and I continued our seminar, and before long I was ready to write.

Meditation Secrets for Women is a synthesis of our discussions. The whole process has been a remarkably seamless and complementary flow between us. I believe these secrets are essential for every woman who wants to meditate, whether you're a seasoned inner traveler or new to the journey. It is my hope that through them you will gain access to more joy and meaning, both in meditation and in life.

Lorin and I are grateful to all the women who have generously revealed their inner world to us. Their stories have fueled and inspired this work.

Camille Maurine
Marina del Rey, California
Summer 2000

Introduction

The sensuous ebb and flow of the breath,
The warmth of the sun on the skin,
The touch of light on the eyelids, like a kiss,
The soothing sound of leaves rustling in the breeze,
The satisfying release of bodyweight into the support of the Earth—
Nothing in particular to do or be,
Just savoring the texture of life in this moment . . .

Relaxing, melting, softening into lusciousness.
Sinking down, letting go, deeper, deeper . . .
Breath spreading, massaging everywhere inside, a gentle caress . . . Ah . . .
Muscles release, a sigh of relief, all the way to the bones.
Here, now, the movement of life, touching me,
Healing me, revealing its simple truth—
I am immersed in the embrace of life.

Yes, I hear the Yes.
And my response, Yes.
I am this movement.
I am home.

෧ ෧ ෧

🙰 COME HOME TO YOURSELF

This is meditation—luxuriating in the sensory world, resting in the simplicity of your own being, enjoying yourself shamelessly.

"What?" you ask. "I thought you had to discipline yourself to meditate. I thought you had to detach from pleasure, override desire, empty the mind." Our response, from more than fifty years of experience between us, is a resounding *no*.

Nature designed us to blossom in the bodily state of pleasure. When we give over to this basic need, every cell, every fiber of body and soul, can receive and come alive. Something way down inside—that primitive place underneath our everyday human personality—is met and satisfied. Touched and fed with pleasure, something awakens, like an animal purring into health and power, or a tender plant blossoming into glorious vibrant color.

The simple pleasure of being completely at home in the body puts us in rapport with the ongoing rhythms of nature. We have a tangible sense of ourselves as an organism within the larger natural environment—connected, contained, safe. As we relax in enjoyment within ourselves, we feel free to release, deep inside, into a condition of easy flow. The pulsings of breath and blood slow into a soothing dance. Our senses dilate; we feel closer to the processes of life.

This openness to the touch of life is at once deeply healing and nutritive. The body opens up to receive, and we are informed—informed—by the vast, fecund, life-giving natural world. And we know:

Life is here. I am here. I am alive.

🙰 Your meditation time is the perfect place to cultivate this natural connection. It may seem like an indulgence, a luxury, but such connection is a vital necessity. For women to be healthy in meditation, their practice must be based in this primary sense of pleasure. No denial of the body, of the instincts, of emotion, your meditation should be a deeply intimate relationship with yourself, with breath, with life. Deep pleasure is like a stem leading down into your feminine roots, connecting you to the rich, fertile ground of being and drawing life force back up so that your individual essence can bloom. With pleasure at its foundation, your meditation is a coming to your senses, a coming home.

Meditation is time carved out for yourself—sacred space—to feel that underlying yes from life, the affirmation of your being. In this spacious welcoming, you may feel the yes of your own response to life welling up from the depths—not from discipline but from pleasure, not from demand but from love.

An Invitation

What woman doesn't yearn for time for herself, without having to be anything for anyone else? To rest, to restore, to settle in. To catch up with all the thoughts that fly in and out all day. To sort out her feelings from the tangle of everyone else's. To be in touch with herself, her body, her rhythm. To clarify her own sense of things. To get back to her essence . . .

We hear about this yearning all the time from the women we work with. But when we mention meditation, resistance rears its head:

- "I want to meditate, but I just don't have the time."
- "I can't sit still, and forget about cross-legged—it hurts my knees."
- "Cleanse my mind of thoughts? Are you kidding?"
- "Be calm and love everybody? Get real. I can't stop the whirring in my head."
- "I don't have the discipline."
- "Meditation's supposed to be good for you, right? But it sounds so dry and boring. I would never want to deny so much of myself."

What if we told you that there really are no odious rules to follow, that meditation is just being yourself? What if we told you that you don't have to change yourself in any way to reap the benefits of meditation?

Well, that's what this book is all about.

The marvelous truth is that you already know how to meditate. We're just here to give you permission to do it—and to do it in your own unique way. If you set up favorable conditions, meditation happens spontaneously. This book is about how to set up those conditions for yourself. Providing a rest deeper than sleep, meditation is refreshing and rejuvenating. It's good for your health, enables you to better deal with stress, and helps you live in harmony with your world. Hundreds of scientific studies have mapped out these beneficial effects. But you'll receive these benefits most fully if you figure out a female way that works *for* your own life, not against it.

There is one sobering but ultimately liberating truth that you need to understand right off the bat. The ancient meditation techniques were not designed for women's bodies and psyches. For years Lorin and I have asked, "What is a female-savvy approach to meditation? Why do some women flourish in meditation while others languish or quit?"

In listening to women talk about their meditation experience, we have both consistently heard and seen that women are natural meditators. Given the chance, they settle into deep meditation and stay there for quite a while, even if they have never meditated before. Lorin has discovered that many people spontaneously invent meditation techniques and practice them for years with very good results—often unwittingly re-creating those in the classic texts. Likewise, many women have come to work with me because they want to explore in an embodied mode through subtle sensing and movement. As we stretch their understanding of what meditation can be, they enter profound and transforming states of awareness.

What's the bottom line? Women need a different kind of meditation approach. Meditation should be joyful, sensuous, engaged, alive. It should be rooted in pleasure. Every woman needs a handful of techniques, not just one. The old rigid time frames, rules about immobility, and devices for blocking feeling deny a woman her basic rights to crave, taste, and experience life as she truly does. Women live right inside the natural rhythms of life—an emotional and physical connection that must be honored and satisfied.

In *Meditation Secrets for Women,* we invite you to use meditation as a way to connect with that natural rhythm, not contort it, and as a way to embrace yourself and all of your experiences, whatever mood you're in, without having to deny or push away what's really going on.

The twelve meditation secrets presented here are so simple that they could easily be overlooked. Why is the value of deep pleasure for women such a secret? It is a state so natural and fundamental, so life-affirming, that you would think we would all celebrate it, almost take it for granted, accepting it as second nature or, in fact, as the first nature it really is. Many of us find it difficult to allow ourselves to dwell in that most basic and nurturing of states. As if we need permission! As if the world will fall apart if we let go. As if we will be stoned to death or burned at the stake if we give in to our natural sensuality.

When we relax into ourselves with pleasure, we eventually encounter deep-seated cultural taboos against enjoying our sensuality, against loving our bodies, against resting in our feminine selves. We run into the hidden judgment that these acts are hedonistic, selfish, base, naughty, shallow, frivolous, or sinful. (Care to supply your own adjectives?) So when you meditate, you will probably have to face those taboos—all the control structures that you've been taught as a woman. All your judgments and criticisms about yourself are sure to surface too. The beautiful thing about meditation is that it gives you the chance to rest in your own nature and to learn to celebrate it.

Enter *Secrets* as you might a doorway into a world you've always longed to find and suspected was there all along. And please, please, come as you are. Don't feel you have to change or "improve" yourself— you don't have to be reverent, you don't have to be serious. Come any way you are at the moment: curious, laughing, tired, rebellious, loving, grumpy, nervous, playful, buzzing with energy, or sleepy. Come on in. Step into this wide-open embrace. Welcome all of who you are, from the small to the vast, the tender to the wise, the mundane to the divine. You'll find that meditation nourishes your heart, and like a visit to an inner therapist, a quick vacation, an emotional tune-up, or a magic healing treatment, it's an experience from which you'll emerge more whole and real and empowered to be your best self.

A Healthy Approach

So here we are in the modern world, where millions of people from every walk of life are meditating every day, and far fewer than 1 percent of them are monks. More than half of all meditators are female: athletes, businesswomen, teachers, students, artists, singers, therapists, actors, moms, kids, and healers of all kinds. Women have become part of the spiritual equation, not just as followers and devotees but as teachers and leaders. Yet, of the thousands of books on meditation, the vast majority are by men from within the various monastic paths. In general, the meditative traditions of the world have perpetuated the following ideas:

Better to sit still than to dance.

Better to be desireless than to have desires.

Better to be detached than to be involved.

Better to be compassionate than passionate.

Better to be aloof than to love.

Better to be obedient than defiant.

Better to submit than to be independent.

Better to follow the tried-and-true path than to find your own.

Better to kill your ego than to live your individuality.

Better to be empty than full.

Better to be male than female.

Monks take vows of celibacy, poverty, and obedience, and so of course their meditation practice is intended to strengthen their ability to live out these vows; any contrary impulses must be crushed. Monasticism and meditation are often confused, but in fact they have little to do with each other. In his talks, the Dalai Lama consistently voices this wisdom, which we heartily celebrate: "Don't be a monk, don't be a Tibetan. Be in your own life and religion. Just meditate, be happy, and have compassion for all beings."

A meditation technique is a way of dealing with your thoughts, emotions, senses, and attention that fosters a deep and peaceful state of repose. When it works, it can lead to an inner harmony that is wonderfully revitalizing. What happens, though, when you impose someone else's technique on yourself? What happens if you impose a style or "mental software" on yourself that was designed for a different kind of person with a different purpose? You usually end up confused to some extent and feeling like a failure.

In our conversations Lorin and I talked more about TM, which I had learned in 1972. He had studied Transcendental Meditation with Maharishi and taught the technique from 1970 to 1975. Lorin reflected on the distinction that Maharishi made: there is a dramatic difference between the path of the recluse or monk and that of the householder. "He made it clear to me that householders—people who live in the world—evolve through the adventure of following their passions, daring to be attached, tolerating great intimacy, and dealing with the ever-changing structure of their relationships. The householder path is to get in touch with your inner peace for half an hour in meditation in the morning, then go out and be dynamic and actively work to make the world a better place. Always, in teaching, he instructed us to give people ways of meditating that support their aspirations and their duties, not ones that may undermine them. If you are working with a business-woman, give her techniques that help her be calm and happy in action. Encourage her ambition."

Another of Maharishi's insights was that one of the worst things you can do as a teacher is to tell people who have busy minds that they have to stop thought. They'll just get tied up in knots, struggling with their own dynamism—a battle they can't win. This insight goes against the age-old stereotype of meditation—that it involves making your mind perfectly still. This may be possible if you live in a cave or a religious order and your life is simplified to the extreme: you live in isolation, don't have a job, don't handle money, don't have dreams, and just follow orders. If you live in the world, love people, feel passionately, and work, you cannot and should not try to impose stillness in meditation. It works much better to embrace motion, including the movement of emotion and thoughts. This kind of meditation gives you a sense of stillness-in-motion. It may last only a few seconds or minutes in your meditation, but it is there and you have touched it.

Women's bodies and psyches have special needs and strengths. For us to be healthy in meditation it must take into account our:

- Body rhythms and hormonal fluctuations
- Emotional complexity and sophistication
- Home base in relatedness
- Intuition
- Natural sensuality
- Multitasking ability
- Deep connection to the cycles of life

New research into women's physiology, sometimes called "liberation biology," is playing a significant role in validating these attributes. Recent studies reveal structural differences between male and female brains, for example, and imaging shows that women tend to use both hemispheres to process information. Such findings suggest a biological base for a woman's access to the unconscious, emotional awareness, and a broader view of life based in connectedness.

Women's nervous systems are already highly responsive; we do not need rigorous practices to make us so. Much more crucial to women is having meditation as a safe sanctuary to process and integrate this sensitivity. Women do not repress the way men do, and our inner reality is different. This should be celebrated, not shamed or feared.

When these differences are not acknowledged in meditation techniques, it cheats women of the benefits. You can injure yourself in meditation, just as you can in running or dancing, when rigid techniques are imposed on you. Meditation brings you to a profound state in which you touch the depths where you are being re-created. You are installing a certain quality in the subtle energy circuits (or *nadis*) of your nervous system. So if you impose repression, it goes deep. Relaxation is sensual, even sexy and electric. But because many women are mentally focused on the guru and the rules, they edit out their natural vigor. As a result, they may be calm during and after meditation but end up devitalized and pale. Meditating in a female-friendly way gives a woman a healthy sense of self and enables her to know who she is from deep within herself. That connection to her core is precious, and not to be denigrated.

As a woman who positively thrives in meditation, I can tell you that it is one of my favorite things to do. Over the years I have joyfully studied several of the ancient methods—TM, esoteric yoga, Zen, and Tibetan Buddhism. I feel deeply akin to those spiritual cultures and cherish their techniques, but I have come to realize that living as an American, in the twenty-first century, in a female form, is a very different experiment in consciousness. The more I have let go of the rigidity of outer structures and learned to listen within, the healthier I have felt. I have come to trust the current of vibrancy that flows through me and informs me of the practice I need each day—always responsive to the movement of my life, and always deeply balancing.

One morning Lorin was in the kitchen feeding the cat when I came out from the bedroom. I had been up past midnight teaching a performance group and was grumpy, tired, and bedraggled. My hair was sticking out at all angles, and that's how I felt inside. I muttered, "I think I'm premenstrual," and after making a cup of tea, I disappeared back into the bedroom to meditate. When I emerged half an hour later, Lorin looked at me and said, laughing, "Amazing, how you do that. Now you look serene, smooth, and refreshed, as if you'd spent the day at a health spa."

"Serene? Ha! I spent the first five minutes growling, hissing, and shaking. In the next five, my breath changed to sobs. Then for ten minutes more my body hummed and swayed with the currents of electricity. And the last few minutes I just sat there with my eyes open, smiling with dangerous glee. I'm more like a wild animal than serene. But I do feel all of one piece, my fur is smoothed out, and I have to admit, I am definitely refreshed!"

Lorin said, "You know, I've seen you work that magic on every mood and circumstance, day in and day out, year after year." We'd been together fifteen years at that point. "But what you do when you meditate," he continued, "is not on the maps. It would surprise a lot of people. Growling? Sobbing? That doesn't sound very detached!" Lorin broke up in laughter. "It's such a female approach, and so healthy—you are not repressing anything." I knew what he meant: this sensual, instinctive vibrancy is just not what most people picture when they think of meditation.

Many women cry during meditation. If you're likely to cry during movies, you will cry in meditation, because it gives you a chance to let your heart melt, to surrender to all the love that you feel. Crying is not even mentioned in most meditation books, yet this complete melting is a way of transcendence through the heart. Life itself is the great teacher. If you are looking at someone or something with total adoration—a pet, or a baby, or your lover—in that moment you are not being egotistical. You have a sense of being part of something larger. You feel connected. In and out of love, we learn about the ego. The realm of the personal leads to the transcendent because all relationships change and create a tug inside our hearts to the extent that we are involved. Pay attention to that movement of change, and you are instantly in meditation.

When women adapt meditation to fit their individuality, the little modifications they make seem like just "common sense" or "a hunch." Women are shy about sharing these tips, which do not feel like wisdom to them; on the contrary, the women we have spoken to often feel ashamed about not being able to fit themselves into the program.

One afternoon in the early 1980s Lorin was sitting in the cafeteria at Esalen, a seminar center perched on a cliff overlooking the Pacific Ocean in Big Sur, California. He was there alone, having a cup of coffee, and there were only a couple of other people in the whole place, although it had seats for over a hundred. A beautiful woman came and sat next to him. From the way she moved, and the way she held her cup of coffee, he could see that she had done a lot of awareness practice—every move she made was full of grace. Striking up a conversation, she asked him what he was doing at Esalen, and he told her he was teaching meditation. She said, very brightly, that she did Zen: she and her husband were very involved in a Zen center and had been "sitting" for years.

Following a hunch, Lorin gently asked, "Don't you think Zen is bad for women? All that sitting still and suppressing the urge to move? Where is the rhythm?"

The woman flinched for a second, as if she had been slapped by an invisible hand. Then, in a testament to her Zen practice, she recovered in a heartbeat and took advantage of the moment. She leaned forward and told him the following story.

"Last year the women—the wives—at the Zen center started getting together each week to talk and have tea. Over time we realized that many of us were having health problems of various sorts, and we wondered what was going on. I mean, we all eat health food and meditate. Our lives aren't particularly stressful. Finally, one woman in the group said, 'You know, I feel like my energy gets activated by the meditation, but then it doesn't get to move. It just stays there and stagnates as we sit there for long hours. I feel like I need to move, to dance the energy.' That rang a bell with many of the other women. We had been doing hours and hours of sitting meditation for years."

Lorin asked, "Did you talk to the teacher about it?"

She said, "Several of us went to talk to the roshi about this, but he brushed us off. We went back to the larger group of women and decided among ourselves to minimize the time we spent sitting and to do walking meditation as our practice. We have been doing this for almost a year, and it seems to be working."

"Did you tell your husbands about it?" he asked.

"No, our husbands are so earnest. And since the teacher rejected our idea, it would just make trouble."

We have heard many such stories, in which women who love meditation adapt it to fit their needs. They find ways to juice it up, to personalize and enjoy it. But often their creativity is scorned by their (mostly male) teachers. Even though the women's methods work and their ideas are practical and helpful, they are treated as heretics. Or they are told that it is "just their ego talking" and that they should surrender more. Consequently, women's precious insights about meditation have not been gathered and used to improve teaching methods, especially methods used to teach women. Every woman has to discover, through trial and error, what works for her and what leads her into stagnation. This process can take many years.

Lorin worked with another woman, Cynthia, who had for seven years been doing a form of Buddhist meditation with very strict rules and fierce visualization practices. She had started meditating at twenty-two, and she was now twenty-nine. After several sessions, having talked for hours about her experiences, she finally said, with considerable fear and trepidation, "Do you think it is possible . . . that these practices . . . were never designed for women?" It had taken Cynthia years of exploration, suffering, wonder, anguish, and soul-searching to get to the point where she could say that. She had been trying to do the practices exactly as taught, in the mood and tone the teacher was putting forth, and she had found that she was having to delete more and more of herself in order to fit the program. "I love meditation, but I don't think these rules apply to people like me."

Monastic notions of "destroying the ego," "detaching from desire," and "killing the instincts" have little relevance to ordinary lives, especially women's lives. These ideas are inappropriate and even harmful. The demands of work, family, and love put great strains on a woman's ego. In meditation we should be looking to strengthen, not weaken, the ego. Ditto desire. We've been trained to detach from our desires for hundreds if not thousands of years. Ditto our instincts. It's time to reclaim them all. And there's no reason on earth not to use our meditation time to do so.

We should give thanks to the lamas, yogis, and roshis for preserving and disseminating the teachings of old. Responding to the global cry for help, they are generously and courageously sharing their path to peace. They've left their monasteries, traveled far from their own countries, and learned our language; they have met us more than halfway. But we cannot expect them to have a clue about female wisdom; that is and has been for women to discover and develop. As women, it is our job to stand on our own ground, in our own bodies, and to adapt meditation to the needs of our lives.

Women have learned all kinds of mantras and techniques, and they've taken vows and followed gurus, but it is their adaptations and integrations that have brought power and beauty to their meditation. They have found ways to meditate that really suit them but haven't told anybody about them. We consider this sacred knowledge. We wrote this book to gather what we could of the hints, discoveries, and insights about meditation that women have revealed to us. We consider it a progress report. The story of women and meditation will undoubtedly take decades to unfold as women meditators and teachers share their experiences. The point is to get and keep the conversation going.

We invite you to dabble, to experiment and find what works best for you. With these secrets in hand, you should be well on your way to falling in love with a style of meditating that works for your body, your needs, and your female mode of being in the world.

Take a deep breath, right now—the kind you take in joy or satisfaction. Ah . . . there, you've already begun.

❧ THE CALL TO REMEMBER

The forces that work against a woman's essential nature are formidable and, sad to say, deeply internalized. I feel it in myself and in women all around me, liberated though we may be. We have cleared a lot of ground; let's celebrate that. We have more freedom, more voice, more power; we know more about what we want and how to go for it. Brava, Brava! Why is it then that creative, intelligent, self-aware women everywhere are silently suffering, finding it almost impossible to endorse themselves, to love their bodies as they are, to luxuriate in the simplicity of being?

The need for embodied internal resources has never been greater. It is certainly *not* a secret that life is becoming ever more complex and unpredictable; there is hardly time to assimilate all the change that is happening, personally and globally. Most of us are deeply concerned about the environment, education, the care of children, indigenous cultures, and endangered species, and we take what action we can. But what about our own nature, our inner environment? It too is endangered. Can we value it just as much?

Bellies and breasts are screaming, trying to get our attention, trying to bring us home.

Just to take time for ourselves, apart from the many relationships we have, can seem almost forbidden. Our lives are so full and complex, with so much to attend to, that the thought of having time to "just be" seems indulgent and impractical. The texture of time itself has become a crunch, rather than a spacious opportunity to unfold. As women, caretakers of the world, we submit our instincts to the needs we read in others. We lose touch with our nature. It is sometimes even foreign to us. We think we must earn entry to the "kingdom" when in fact the land is free, and right beneath our feet.

There is the stress of heroically making our way in an increasingly demanding atmosphere. Most women juggle many roles, trying to hold body and soul together for self and loved ones. We also have the psychic burden of carrying feelings for our world, our immediate situation as well as the larger global context. Women tend to perceive and process any emotional subtext that isn't being addressed—overwhelming—but, hey, somebody's gotta do it! Then we have the challenging transformations of maturing—okay, aging—and the cultural shame attached to that process. No matter what our age or shape, there is always some ideal, sleekly marketed image to compare ourselves to. Insidious! If we manage not to condemn ourselves, it's usually only after a long struggle. And just to ride the fluctuations of hormones, the physical and emotional cycles we all have, while tending to the needs of children, relationships, and work . . . how do we do it all?

Women work so hard, inside and out; many of us are more exhausted than we know. Depression—that inner pull down and in—seems almost epidemic among women today. Why? Let's face it, our feminine roots are calling us. Our bodies and psyches are starving for that deeper nourishment. Without it, we cannot thrive. Without it, something essential dies, sacrificed on the altar of masculine values and power.

It's ironic, isn't it, that something so fundamental and natural should require such conscious tending. But . . . it does. In this wildly demanding and precarious world, we need the foundation of our feminine roots—big-time.

We must "re-mind" each other. We must remember, again and again.

Break the Shame

When we enter the territory of pleasure and sensuality, we come up against the tyranny of cultural attitudes about the body. In spite of all our supposedly enlightened attitudes, we are still pretty confused. Pleasure, or sensuality, is not valued just for itself—for ourselves. One way or another, it becomes contrived, complicated, foreign—somehow not ours.

As women, we've become used to seeing ourselves as an object, making ourselves into a project, or marketing ourselves one way or another. It's so easy to believe that something is wrong with us, that we have to fix this or that about ourselves to find acceptance. Our sense of self is packaged, evaluated, priced, and sold at the market of social expectations. Is it ever enough? Our sensuality, or internal value, gets all mixed up with desirability, or external value. And how easily our sensuality is sexualized, appropriated to serve something else, or some*one* else. Rather than being in pleasure, we try to become pleasing. The fragile flame of self-worth flickers in the cultural wind.

Most women feel a subtle (or not so subtle) shame for never living up to the collective ideals about the body and about sexuality. We try to fit some image that we think will bring us love—you know the story all too well. Of course, we can never measure up.

Ideals of perfection split us off from ourselves. We feel fragmented, somehow never quite right. Cut off from our own deeper impulses, we come to mistrust them. We forget the natural sensuality and deep-body knowing that could be our anchor and our strength.

In truth, our whole culture seems to be grappling with these issues today. Health and fitness have become more highly valued, but paradoxically, that very body awareness, instead of cultivating internal well-being, has fueled the quest for just the right look, the right shape, the right tone of sexy appeal. We are in a collective trance, searching with religious zeal for the new Holy Grail—the perfect body.

Images of women, beautiful and free, constantly bombard us through the media—TV, movies, magazines. The very images that purport to be liberating for women are alienating, distorting, and imprisoning. More often than not the women in these images are rail-thin with bionic breasts—an unlikely combination. This is not news. But admit it: even though you know better, how many idealized images do you carry around in your head of models and movie stars, and how often do you judge yourself against them?

We are so used to the game, the competition, the sense of inadequacy, the envy of or from other women. The blade can cut both ways. Even when someone pays us a compliment, we find it hard to receive it. Don't be too happy, too full, too okay—as though we must apologize for our own blossoming. There's always something to chop us down or push us back. A friend says, "Hey, you're lookin' good!" and you feel like saying, "No, really?" (*I don't believe her. Why is she saying that? What does she want?*) So you respond, "Yeah, well, you should see me when I wake up in the morning!" Or there we are with a lover who is caressing and adoring us, and all we can think of is, *Oh, God, my lumpy thighs, my sagging boobs!*

It is big business to play on the insecurities of women, and commercial fortunes are made as they flit around from one cosmetic solution to another. Aging has many women terrorized and in dread. The hypnosis of cultural attitudes has formidable power. We repeat the lines like catechism: *I am not worthy, I am not worthy.* It is a mighty challenge to break the spell.

To stay centered in oneself, at home in your own body in the midst of this onslaught, can seem like a Sisyphean task. If you're a baby-boomer, as I am, you may have noticed some inevitable changes in the mirror. There are so many of us, however; my hope is that we will bust right through the trance—strength in numbers, you know. So take heart, you are not alone. We're in this together, and we are learning to set ourselves free.

Feminism and Sensuality

You would think that feminism had addressed the issues I'm raising here, but strangely enough, women's sensuality has become almost a politically incorrect topic these days. Feminism originated as an affir-mation of woman as subject, not object. It was about women asserting their own power and striving for freedom and equality with men. But pleasure is often a casualty of feminism—or perhaps a misapplication or misunderstanding of it. Let there be no mistake: to live from your foun-dation in deep pleasure is a political act of power.

Power in the world is still associated primarily with masculine val-ues. Women who work hard, have careers, and are intelligent and socially aware often seem to fear their own feminine nature. Don't say we're different from men—we'll lose the ground we've gained! Being sensual feels too fluffy, too vulnerable, too much like being a bimbo. How will anyone take us seriously? Or women are so exhausted from being on the front lines that they feel they've run out of time and ener-gy for such silly, trivial self-indulgence. *If I relax and let down,* the mod-ern woman wonders, *will I ever get up again?*

Sensuality can feel dangerous and unmanageable. If we give over to it, our world could become too sexualized, we might not be able to get our jobs done or keep the professional respect we need, and meeting people could become a messy ordeal. And we might have to deal with all the emotions that being in touch with ourselves brings up. We'd bet-ter just keep our sensuality under wraps.

Once again we are split off from deep pleasure—the body-based, feminine home in ourselves.

A woman I'll call Sharon poignantly articulated this common dilemma. After attending several classes, she had come to private sessions, saying, "In these classes I'm discovering something about being a woman, and I want to go deeper." A skilled writer in her forties, Sharon works in a high-pressure job and is very concerned about social issues. She's been practicing Buddhist meditation for years. The mental clarity and simplicity of those forms appeal to her, and like many women, she deals with the patriarchal structure by thinking of it as androgynous. But after speaking for a while, she admitted that her woman self often feels metaphorically locked away in a cellar, screaming and flailing against the door.

Deep down Sharon feels lusty, vibrant, and passionate, qualities immediately apparent in her movement. But because she finds it difficult to manage her intensity and she experiences deep pain from thwarted desire (especially in relationships), it is not easy for her to stay in touch with that aspect of herself. She describes her body as voluptuous, but since she associates voluptuousness with vulnerability, she camouflages herself in baggy clothes to avoid "advertising" it. And though she longs for a relationship, she also seems to have given up on it. Sharon has done years of therapy and is also on Prozac, yet low-level depression still lurks in the background of her awareness. As she spoke, she realized with grief that her woman self has stopped crying out for acknowledgment and has gone mute in disappointment.

Through breathwork and movement, Sharon reconnected to the freedom, power, and joy of her feminine nature—and her tenderness. We laughed, cried, and hooted together as she danced her revelations. Recently I asked her to consider letting a smidgen of her sensuality come into her sitting meditations—even just for a minute—as an experiment. I could sense her hesitation. "In the business world you learn to contain your sensuality, and it's the same at the meditation center. You just accept that that's the way it is." But she recognized the vibrancy and power of letting her sensuality flow through her body as life force. "That is true and possible and probably a lot more healthy and generous to oneself. I hope that I can return to it before I'm too old." So she laughed and replied that maybe she could stay for a few minutes after the regular meditation period at the center.

Over these many years I have worked with thousands of women who hear the call into their deep feminine wisdom. Some are just beginning the journey; others are well versed in exploration. They are women of every age, from pubescent to postmenopausal. All of them struggle with the ideals that fragment the female psyche and separate them from their bodies, instincts, and emotional truth.

I would like to think that younger women are less susceptible to this internal split, but confusion about bodies, sensuality, and sexuality seems just as pervasive as ever. Ironically, thanks to our more liberal social posture, girls must now navigate through even more conflicting images and behaviors as they try to find some sense of self. Teenage eating disorders, cutting of the flesh, and other self-destructive symptoms are the cries of that struggle. May we heed those cries and respond with our own hard-won wisdom.

In this book we offer some tools for remembering—the secrets of how to meditate from the roots of your being. Meditation works *for* you, in the service of your life. It is not just time out; it is time in. Come home to your body, to your own nature, to the richness of your senses. Be subject, not object. Meditation will then enrich all of your relationships and nourish you so that you can more fully engage in your world with instincts intact.

You already have moments of this connection. Simple pleasures that you love are doorways into this broader body knowing, this fundamental ground of being that is always there, under the surface, waiting to be felt. Life is generous: given the slightest opening, it comes gushing through.

Each time that ground of being is touched with your awareness, something grows. Each and every time you remember, a substance accrues, the essence of your being. As it grows stronger and more tangible, you begin to live and move and breathe in the experience of being. Slowly and surely, you find yourself in a new body, the living reality of the body of love.

Your Secret

As you cultivate the sense of pleasure, you can let it be your little secret. What happens in meditation is contained within the privacy of your inner world. Nobody has to know what you are experiencing inside yourself, so set yourself free. People will wonder why you have that strange smile playing around your lips. Let them wonder; you'll never tell.

✌ WHAT WOMEN EXPERIENCE IN MEDITATION

Body Awareness

"I'm aware of the tension in my muscles, little aches all over my body, particularly in my neck, shoulders, and back. When I realize I don't have to hold myself up now or be on duty, it starts to let go."

"My body relaxes. Deeper breaths start to happen naturally. I feel more spacious and free, sometimes as big as the galaxy."

"It is as though a balm flows all over my skin. It smoothes me out and soaks into my pores."

"Warm, billowy waves of pleasure."

"A delicate internal touch, like rose petals on my inner skin."

"I sense life coursing through me. There is a tingle and a hum."

"I feel at home in myself, in my body, and in my life."

Thoughts

"I'm always aware of the long list of things I have to do. I think about my challenges, situations I have to show up for. I replay recent interactions with people and sort out my experience."

"A higher perspective gradually emerges. . . . I see the whole swirling movement of my life, but rather than being 'outside' and caught up in it, I am centered inside it."

"It gives me time to remember the bigger picture, being part of the world, nature, and the universe. This takes me into wonder about the miracle of creation, and the mystery of what it is to be a human being."

Emotions

"I begin to notice all the background emotions I could sense were there but haven't had time to process. Often I cry, or realize I'm angry about something and need to speak up. As I feel through all this, I reconnect with my core."

"I'm aware of all the suffering, of people I know who are going through painful times, someone in emotional crisis or in the hospital, and the violence and oppression throughout the world. But it opens my heart and makes me feel close to them. I send out love and healing energy, and sometimes I discover surprising ways I can take action to help."

"I take a pause to appreciate aspects of my life, everything I love and value, the richness of my personal connections. It is inspiring, like listening to beautiful music, and I am filled with gratitude."

"I sense currents of energy that are exciting, soothing, luscious, cleansing, nourishing, reorganizing, and balancing. It's always a different mix of these elements."

"Each breath feels like it flushes my system. It's like being washed and rinsed with free-flowing emotional energy."

"The cobwebs in the corners have been swept clean."

"Everything inside gets to shift around and find its right place. There is more clarity, like when the sand settles to the bottom of a lake."

"I let go so deeply it's as if I'm asleep, but I'm not. Images float by like in a dream. It's better than the drugs I used to take. Sometimes I get great creative ideas for a project I'm working on."

"When I meditate, I feel like I'm being cared for, like I'm 'having my nerves done,' or getting a massage. Afterwards I feel together, as if I'm wearing the right clothes and my hair looks good."

"I get to catch up to all the conversations that I've missed. I can hear myself think. I get to feel how much love is in my heart for all my family and friends. I end up feeling perfectly poised in the center of my world. I always get there even though I have to listen to ten minutes of inner chatter first. I think it will never end, then it surprises me and goes silent."

"When I simply make time for myself, it's as though the presence of life is right there waiting and eager to feed me. I can let it penetrate me, sink in and saturate me. I absorb it by just being aware."

Let your meditation be a place to break the rules, whatever they have been for you. This may be in defiance of every expectation you have of meditation. We all have some kind of inhibition against our own pleasure, wildness, and joy. Challenge those taboos. Embrace your sensuality. Break free of that old shame.

Perhaps for you it will be the feeling of having a beautiful inner sanctuary, a place of refuge just for you. Or it may be an inner knowing, a sense of being part of the movement of nature, an intuitive but tangible connection to the fertility of life and your own place within it. You may reconnect with the primitive, wild animal power inside you, as though your skin is covered in lustrous fur, your whiskers twitching, and your eyes alert. It may be the experience of having a Divine Lover who sees you and adores you just as you are, who holds and caresses you exactly the way you like. Or your sensuality may even feel like an illicit pleasure, as if you are having a steamy, passionate affair—but the affair is with life itself! Whatever you discover, savor the feeling. Accept it. Let it teach you. Walk around the world with that luscious secret living inside you, your own personal mystery.

This intimacy with ourselves is essential for us as women. It is the ground, the foundation for every other relationship in our lives. Even a minute here and there can make a huge difference. Indulge yourself. You will emerge rejuvenated and renewed. Then you can share that gift in the relationships of your life, from a place of being full within yourself. It's your choice. So come on in! Enjoy yourself, shamelessly.

❧ AT HOME IN HERSELF

The writer Alice Walker shows us how natural meditation can be. "When I was a child, I felt so much a part of the countryside and everything that was in it that I couldn't avoid the feeling that I had to have been loved very much, to find myself there.

"So when I came to meditation—I actually started doing TM when I was living in New York after a divorce—it was a kind of going back. Just after being initiated in doing the training, when I finally sort of got it, I started to laugh, because I recognized where I was. I was back in a place where I had lived as a child, in my spirit, in a very open, spacious, loving place, where I felt totally at peace and in myself."

❧ SOME IDEAS ON HOW TO USE THIS BOOK

A book on meditation is just a collection of hints—the real skills are always learned from the inside. The adventure here is to find your own secrets—ways to be with yourself in meditation that match your individual nature and the needs and desires of your own life. Meditation is an embrace of your entire being, with no judgment—and we all need help with that.

Use this book as a support in caring for yourself. In a thousand different ways meditation is self-care. It is tendering unto, attending to, the soul, the spirit, and the body. Think of your "self" as the integration of all levels of your being. Be self-ish. You do not have to be religious to meditate, but meditation can complement and deepen your prayers. You may have heard the old saying, "Prayer is talking to God. Meditation is listening." You do not even have to consider yourself spiritual. In fact, your bad, bawdy, irreligious self may be just the key. Over time meditating does expand the lens of perception, and you may be surprised by an ineffable new connection to creation, the universe, or the source of life, a sense of your place within the whole.

The twelve secrets are presented in twelve chapters, each of which includes exercises designed to be done easily and comfortably in the midst of your daily life. As you read and do the explorations, notice the response in your body. Don't worry about "doing it right." Just go with what works well with your body and feelings today.

Each chapter includes:

- *Explorations:* questions for you to muse and write about that help to personalize the material. There is also a "Warm-up" for you to play with to get the gist of an aspect of meditative experience. These are fun experiments in awareness that will come in handy later.

- *Skill Circle:* practical tips to build the skills that will enrich your experience in meditation. Each skill circle highlights a particular quality of paying attention related to that secret.

- *Meditations:* awareness practices, as well as breath, sound, and simple movement meditations. There are a few to start with, followed by a "Going Further" section that provides more meditations that you can investigate over time. The variety that we offer shows how fecund meditation can be; there are plenty for you to stretch into for many years to come. Take your time. Don't feel you have to do them all; just do the ones that appeal to you now. Start with any one meditation that seems interesting and explore it for a week or so. Let it teach you about that way of paying attention, then return to it occasionally whenever you like. You will also get hints for inventing your own meditations, so go ahead and improvise if you get the urge.

- *Reflections:* questions to help you integrate what you've discovered through that chapter's secret.

In addition, Secret #12 provides some gentle stretches to do before or after meditating. We also recommend that you read a page or two of a secret right before you meditate. New skills are best learned by putting them into practice right away. As the information on the page becomes your own experience, you begin to embody new muscular and neural behaviors—new ways to be alive. Each of the secrets is about accepting the experience you are already having; you just haven't taken the time to notice it, or you haven't opened your senses to that realm.

Instead of working at meditation, play at it. Animals learn new behaviors through play and practice. It's better to be mischievous than serious and sanctimonious. Even while you read, experiment with being natural, spontaneous, and free. The more at ease you are while reading the book, the more effectively what you learn transfers into the physical skill of meditating. The act of reading itself should feel luxurious and fun. If it doesn't, you might ask yourself a few questions: Am I relaxed? Am I breathing easily? Am I furrowing my brow? Am I pushing on to get to the next sentence? Is there something that I don't understand? Do I need to go back and reread anything? Do I need to take a break, go for a walk, take a breath, ponder some question, doubt, or worry?

Consider creating a special *Secrets* journal in which you can write down your responses to the explorations and keep track of experiences from your meditative journey. You could record your night dreams and see whether there is any correlation to your meditative insights. Use words, draw, paint, or snip images from magazines that catch your fancy and paste them in. Externalizing your insights, questions, and musings in this manner honors the fertility of your psyche, which in its generosity will surely reward you with even more revelations.

Get creative about how, when, and where you meditate. Gather a few friends and explore the secrets together; read and discuss any passages that you find useful, controversial, or inspiring. Do a meditation or two together and reflect on your discoveries. There is a synergy, an amplification of energy, when two or more are gathered. This creates not only a stronger field of attention but also moral support for a feminine approach and affirmation for forging your individual style. As you swap notes with each other, you're exercising your voice and developing a new language for feminine experience. It is always fascinating to discover our idiosyncrasies as well as commonalties within a group of women. Group energy is especially potent with the movement and sound experiments—which are very liberating and sometimes highly entertaining.

The most important thing is that you find the gifts that each secret holds for you and make them your own, incorporating them into your meditation in your own way. Each offers insights that will enhance your experience in the others. As time goes on, you will probably cycle through them all. Some of the secrets may not ring any bells right now, or you may already have them under your belt. But one of the secrets will be your current cutting edge. Pick up whatever colorful strands appeal to you and weave them together into your own special fabric of meditation.

❧ COMMON QUESTIONS

When is the best time to meditate?

Meditation is usually most helpful before periods of activity—in the morning and again in the afternoon or early evening. By meditating at these times, you carry the relaxation of meditation out into your daily life. If you meditate before bed, keep it short—five or ten minutes only.

How long do I meditate each time?

There is a natural body rhythm of a twenty-minute rest cycle, so that is a good amount of time to meditate. Give yourself several minutes to settle in and to come back out slowly. You can also grab one- to five-minute meditations here and there throughout your day.

What posture is best?

Postures are recommended with each of the meditations in this book, but in general, sitting in whatever position you find comfortable is best. You do not have to sit cross-legged. Some people with back problems like to meditate lying down.

Do I have to slow down?

No. Let your mind move as fast as it wants.

What if I think the entire time?

For people with busy lives, meditation often feels that way. Accept your thoughts and keep coming gently back to the focus.

How much effort do I make in meditation?

Slightly less than the effort of moving your eyes to read this sentence.

What about outside noise?

There is almost always outside noise, but it is not a problem. Think of it as the music of life. It is part of the rhythm of meditation to hear outside sound and then return to the focus.

What if I fall asleep?

Almost everybody has a sleep deficit, so most people nod off for a few minutes in every meditation.

What if I am interrupted?

If possible, take a few seconds of transition time before you respond. In general, minimize interruptions by unplugging the phone. You could put a "Do Not Disturb" sign on the door.

Is meditation at all dangerous?

It's about as risky as sitting on your sofa, and probably less dangerous than watching TV.

🎔 THE BASIC STEPS

1. Select one of the meditations at the end of each chapter, or refer to the "Menu of All Meditations" in "Secret #12: Live It Up."

2. Prepare the room. Turn off the ringer of the phone, make sure you have fresh air, and have a blanket or sweater available in case you get cold.

3. Find a comfortable position and posture, as suggested in the meditation.

4. Take two or three minutes to settle in. Just be aware of yourself, noticing what you are feeling.

5. Begin the meditation procedure, gently becoming interested in the focus, whether it is a sensation, an image, or a sound.

6. As is natural, your mind will drift. At times you will be with the focus, then your attention will wander. Just keep coming back to the focus, gently, without judging yourself for wandering. The movement of attending to the focus, drifting, then returning is the primary rhythm of meditation.

7. After fifteen or twenty minutes, let go of the focus and just be with yourself comfortably.

8. Sit for at least three minutes, letting your body and senses reorient to the world. Then open your eyes slowly. Move your fingers and hands, wiggle your toes. Stretch.

9. Gradually make the transition to your regular active state.

Keep your practice simple: there is no need to make up rules or to borrow them from elsewhere. For example, you could make up a rule that thoughts have to move slowly, or that certain types of thoughts—angry or sexual ones—are not allowed. This is a waste of time and energy. In meditation your task is simply to witness your experience from a restful place, without judgment.

Over time collect at least three and preferably five or six meditations that match your cravings so that when you go to meditate each day you can meet yourself as you are. You will need to browse to find just the ones meant for you. We have found that people have very good instincts for the kind of meditation they need at a given time. Gaining access to that instinct is part of the preparation for meditation. Even though you may at times feel uncertain—"Who am I to pick my own meditation?"—go ahead and explore.

Just show up for your meditation time. Maybe at first you will spend most of the time reading this book and only a minute here and there doing one of the meditations. Over time, as you gain confidence, you'll spend more of the time with your eyes closed, meditating, referring back to the book only occasionally.

MEDITATION
SECRETS
FOR WOMEN

❧ SECRET #1
CELEBRATE YOUR SENSES

Self-care, yep, I could use some self-care.
A million things to do today, but meditating will help.
Off I go into my Regeneration Chamber . . .

A little lazy, too tired to sit up straight . . .
I'll just prop myself up with lots of pillows all around.
Some music would be good—gentle and nourishing . . .
Yes, that's the perfect ambient sound to feed my soul.

Hmm, have to remember to call the dentist . . .
Stop at the market on my way back from the bookstore.
Oh yeah, and the post office and bank . . .
Okay, okay, may as well spend a minute to choreograph the day,
Then I can relax. . . . Now, what do I want as my focus? What tone do I need?
Comfort and ease . . . yes, just let me bask in pleasure.

Mmm . . . the music caresses me, soothes me like a healing balm.
And my breath is so soft—filling me, billowing me,
Massaging me tenderly inside. How can it be so sweet?
My whole body is washed with sweetness, inside and out . . .
Ahh . . . my heart lifts, spreads open, and smiles.

I breathe the sweetness in, again and again.
So many sensations of joy . . .
Whew, it's almost hard to take!
Now I imagine the course of my day guided by this pleasure.
I take it with me into the world, with that secret smile inside.

❧ ❧ ❧

A FEAST FOR THE SENSES

Although meditating is often thought of as going beyond sensory experience, it is really a journey through the full range of the senses. Our senses bring us into the present moment, and it is only in the present that we can truly receive life's gifts. This ability to be more present is one of the profound benefits of meditation.

Meditation is a *feast* for the senses. It is outrageous and extravagant, like a banquet of exquisite delicacies with the best company, the finest orchestra, the perfect dance partner, the most elegant ambiance, the greatest sense of leisure, the most considerate attendants, and the most expensive wine. It is a state of extreme wealth and luxury in which you are completely saturated in pleasure. It is over-the-top lusciousness that would probably be illegal outside of the privacy of your interior world. But far from harming anyone, it only benefits the world—especially you. As you breathe in this lushness, you open to the gush of life, to how generously life gives you the next breath and fills you with its sustenance.

The pleasure of meditation induces a dilation of the senses. It is a state of heightened appreciation that enhances our ability to see the details of life with fresh eyes. This opens us up to an aesthetic perception of our environment and ourselves—a poetic, nonliteral sensibility that transforms experience. Everyday reality takes on new meaning: we are living inside an ever-unfolding creation of beauty and mystery. This is certainly something to celebrate!

OUTER AND INNER SENSUALITY

In this chapter you will learn how to let your favorite sensory pleasures be the focus for your meditations. There is a loop of enjoyment between the outer pleasure of activity and the inner pleasure of meditation, a positive feedback through which each amplifies and informs the other. Think of some sensuous activities:

- Gardening in the warmth of the sun
- Going barefoot in the grass
- Eating a scrumptious meal
- Grooving to music

- Singing your heart out
- Making love
- Cradling a sleeping child in your arms
- Holding a soft purring cat on your lap
- Taking your dog for a walk
- Riding a horse
- Smelling a rose or gardenia

Each activity has a special tone that is a clue to your health and satisfaction and to your personal meditative style. Meditation can take on these vibrant textures, intensify them, and even augment your appreciation of those very same acts.

The more senses you engage in meditation, the more interesting it is. Let's take a minute for a little experiment. Right here and now, just as you are, sitting or lying there, what feelings of pleasure can you find? What are the little sensory clues that give you that feeling? Maybe there's the cushiness of the couch or chair you're sitting in, providing a sense of comfort or support. Perhaps as you breathe you notice suddenly you want to take a fuller breath, and it feels good. Or you look out into your environment and appreciate something from the colors, shapes, or movement in the world around you. You may smell someone's cooking, or flowers in a nearby vase. Maybe you can hear the voice of someone you love in the next room, or the sound of the wind in the trees outside. Take a few moments to just let yourself drift, enjoying these impressions. Which senses are at play in the pleasure of this moment?

Each sense is a world of wonder that we usually take for granted, and each mode of sensing awakens different parts of the brain. There are many more senses than the five we have been taught to recognize— smell, vision, touch, hearing, and taste. We also have senses for balance, motion, temperature, the position of our joints, the oxygen in our blood, and many fine subtleties of touch. Most activities are actually *synesthesia,* the combination of many senses simultaneously. Dining at a restaurant, for example, involves not just the taste and texture of your food but its presentation, its smell mixed with the other aromas of the place, the decor and the particular ambiance of sounds and movement, your dinner companion and the quality of your conversation. There is also your own *body kinesthesia*—how you reach to take a bite, breathing in the aroma, the act of chewing and leaning back to savor, internal sensations of excitement and satisfaction. Your enjoyment comes from this rich panoply of impressions.

Some of the most profound meditations occur in the presence of great art, music, or performance. In September 1998 my friend Carol and I went on an art safari in New York, saturating ourselves with theater and dance. We also attended the Pierre Bonnard exhibit at the Museum of Modern Art with Carol's mother. As we sauntered through the halls and paused at each painting, there was a palpable atmosphere of appreciation. Bonnard's scintillating colors seemed to penetrate not only into the eyes but into one's entire being. We three sat together and meditated (what else can you call it?) amid the hush and brush of bodies, the murmurs and sighs that approached reverence. Carol and I had the same experience: our bodies percolated with exhilaration as the color pulsed inside us and with the *participation mystique* of this aesthetic communal ritual.

Each sense is an intimate pathway that joins our outer and inner natures. The senses are not just pointed to the outer world but also tell us what is happening in our inner world. It is through interior sensing that we know what we are feeling and thinking. Think of anything from your life today, and you see, hear, and feel that event. Even abstract thinking is internal sensing. Meditation makes use of this ability to generate a thought or to call up an experience. The techniques—even the ancient and esoteric ones—are all sensory experiences. It is a mistaken notion that subtle inward experience is beyond the senses.

Our sensorium is designed to explore the environment through a remarkable range of perception, from the obvious and grand to the barest subtlety. With touch, there is the range between being boldly grabbed and being caressed with exquisite softness and sensitivity. The lightest touch can be the most soulful, the most powerful and penetrating—and exactly what we crave. With the kinesthetic sense, there's the range of motion from dynamic movement all the way to the tiniest muscular shifts. With sight, we can see in both bright sunlight and the dim illumination from the moon or stars at night, and we experience the full spectrum of color, from the intense primaries to the nuances of pastel.

In the same way, we perceive a broad range of internal cues. In meditation we start with the outer world and then follow the path of the senses inward toward our essence. We can honor the craving for soft caress, for example, and then let it extend into the world of progressively more delicate sensation beyond our usual ken until it touches the innermost core of our being. Similarly with sound, our love of outer music can lead us into internal realms of hearing so refined they seem celestial. We can discern inner sound fading away into profound silence and peace. The internal world of sight conveys vivid scenes from memory, dream, or fantasy, beautiful abstract designs and the faintest of spectral images. Likewise, we enjoy the whole continuum of kinesthesia from feeling like dancing wildly to sitting still and detecting the quiet pulsing of our heart. The relaxation of floating in the ocean has an internal counterpart as well: in meditation there are sensations of being immersed and suspended that are like bathing in the source of life.

This is what we mean when we say that meditation is about luxuriating in your own sensuous experience. The richness of sensory awareness bridges your inner and outer pleasure and opens you to the miraculous wealth of living fully in both worlds.

& TIDBITS OF FAVORITE PLEASURE MEDITATIONS

"Sitting on my balcony garden in the sun, I crush a few leaves of lavender or basil in my fingers and inhale their fragrance."

(Carol, psychotherapist and professor)

"Puttering around the house in the morning, humming to myself."

(Jane, TV producer)

"Drinking my morning cappuccino with total gusto."

(Marta, writer)

"Before, during, and after a bath!"

(Sandra, therapist and performer)

"Gardening and being in nature. I have to be outside."

(Jeanne, teacher)

"Lying on a chaise under a big broom bush, gazing up through the leaves into the beautiful New Mexico sky."

(Anna, massage therapist)

"Standing at the water's edge, watching how the light plays on the waves."

(Kathleen, writer)

"I love spaciousness, so I look at the weather. From my house I can see the clouds over the mountains, so I just sit and watch. Or I go for a walk and pay attention to the way the weather is changing."

(Lillian, video artist, writer, and editor)

&8& ACTIVE PLEASURE MEDITATION

Remember the glow, the vitality, the confidence, and the satisfaction from one of your favorite physical activities—for example, hiking, dancing, swimming, singing, working out, or gardening. How do you feel while engaged in that activity? Healthy, mobilized, strong? Sweaty, down and dirty, invincible? Expressive and free? Graceful, in your own flow? What are the pleasurable aftereffects? Muscles tired but deliciously relaxed, the feeling of being well used? Proud of yourself, virtuous? Energized but balanced, in touch with your body?

Take these same impressions into your sitting (or lying down) meditation. Re-create the pleasant feelings and appreciate them in detail. As you remember and embody that state, you bring it into the present. Enjoy how meditation can be internally active and powerful, not only calming and quiet.

&8& WHAT K.T. LOVES

At twenty-nine, K.T. is the youngest executive for an entertainment merchandising company—and the only woman. To prepare for her day, K.T. meditates in bed when she wakes up, contemplating everything she loves.

"During the day I deal with so many stressed-out people trying to pressure and take advantage of me. I work harder than the other executives, but they still bully and deprecate me. I have very good self-esteem and know how to take care of myself, but I have to stay on my toes so I don't take in their negativity. So when I meditate, I create a place to steep myself in everything that's great about life: flowers, cats, my friends, my fiancé. I meditate on the sensory qualities of what I love. In my heart I touch my lover, my kitties; I breathe in the sunlight and ocean air. I see my favorite flowers and imagine their color and fragrance. This attunes my senses to the world that I want to live in and help create.

"Then when I'm at work and in these meetings, seeing people backstab each other and jockey for power, it doesn't cut through me. Staying centered in the beauty and goodness in life gives me strength. When I don't make time to meditate, I really notice it. It's a different day when I take even five or ten minutes."

K.T.'s experience shows how utterly simple and functional your meditation can be—something that really makes a difference in daily life. Because meditation is so natural, it is also easy to forget to do it; it hardly seems like a technique. It is more a way of being with the self than a way of doing or improving the self. A healthy meditation practice builds on these qualities of enjoyment.

PLEASURE AND HEALTH

Lest you think that this celebration of pleasure is merely rhapsodic New Age thinking or poetic waxing in favor of hedonistic indulgence, let us reassure your critical mind that new research supports the value of pleasure to a woman's health.

You can wash stress out of your system by nurturing yourself with pleasure. The Stress Institute in Boulder, Colorado, has determined that when you don't take enough time out to nurture yourself, you weaken your immune system, making yourself more vulnerable to all types of colds, viruses, and flus. Even such simple things as getting your hair done or having a facial or massage can make a difference.

Healthy Pleasures by Robert Ornstein and Dr. David Sobel is chock-full of information about the benefits of pleasure when it comes to your health. "Every human being possesses an effective internal health maintenance system, one guided by pleasure. Indeed, there is good scientific evidence that we are built for pleasure. Deep brain centers respond directly to pleasure sensations." They continue, "Many of us are not getting our minimum daily requirement of sensual pleasure."

So go ahead, pamper yourself in your favorite ways and know that you're taking care of your health. And guess what? You can also meditate for twenty minutes once or twice a day and get the same results; meditation just happens to be one of the very best ways to reduce stress. The meditations we're suggesting—basking in sensuousness—cost you nothing, are available anytime you are, and can take you into even deeper bliss.

MEDITATION AND SEX

The quality of attention in meditation is a lot like sex—when you find the way *you* like it. It is a delicate internal meeting, a meandering discovery of what you enjoy, and a gradual surrender into more and more pleasure. And afterward you feel great! You're a new woman, totally yourself: connected, renewed, juicy, and relaxed.

The process is also very similar in meditation and in sex: in response to an inner urge or call, you give yourself the time and space to explore sensuously. You create the safety to relax. Both meditation and sex are the best when there's no demand for anything in particular to happen. You simply allow yourself to enjoy and gently unfold. You get interested. You focus on the intriguing sensory details, and as you pay attention, your senses are turned on. You become present, and you start to let go. Inevitably, just about then, you suddenly find yourself thinking of something else: *I have to do the laundry*, or, *Uh-oh, I didn't call Suzy back.* You are "away" for a few seconds. But naturally and eventually, the pleasure calls you back (it is a compelling focus), and as you go with the sensations and movement, you let go a little more. There is a slow dilation deep inside, a melting open. You tap into your succulent nature. This cycle happens in waves, deepening in intensity, until you are absorbed in pleasure, taken over by the energy. Currents of life force surge through you, clearing pathways down to your toes and up through the top of your head, revitalizing every cell and balancing everything.

Meditation is a communion with yourself. You are finding what works for you—your rhythm, your body, your emotions. Its gentle, undemanding touch can help to heal any places of trauma, sexual wounding, or inhibition. The secrets you learn in meditation enrich your sensuality within yourself and if you choose to open sexually with another. Meditative awareness can be a rapturous lovemaking with the universe. This secret awaits you.

TABOO CHECK

When we slow down and enjoy our senses, we claim our sensuality. Sensuality can be defined as surrender to voluptuous experience. Meditation stretches you; when you stretch the range of your senses, it feels fabulous. But you will come up against your personal limitations on pleasure. Confront the taboo to pleasure; meet it head-on. Does all this sensuousness sound outrageous, scandalous, or downright wrong? Meditation this earthy may not be what you expected. Does this approach seem counterintuitive to what you've heard about meditation? Let's take a look at this belief.

When you meditate, you enter a special state of relaxation. Physiological research has found that it is a state of rest even deeper than sleep, but you're awake inside. Part of the time you're even watching yourself dream. You may never have rested this deeply before, or been conscious while so relaxed. What does incredible restfulness feel like? What does it feel like to lie in bed or on the beach and be completely at ease? It is delicious; it is sensuous.

Meditation is a distinct state with its own rules and permissions. A major part of learning to meditate is unlearning patterns of stress. You learn not to carry over the rules of work, driving, or school to your internal time with yourself. Work is good, but if you make meditation into work, it won't be respite. It'll just be one more damn chore on your long to-do list. Dispense with the old "no pain no gain" attitude. It is obsolete and untrue. Find your way to stretch a little more in the direction of pleasure. Part of your learning in meditation is to tolerate these new sensations.

Unless you give yourself permission to let meditation be sensuous and voluptuous, you tend to limit your range. You miss half the experience and half the benefits. Women have a natural sensuality and, unless interfered with, tend to experience meditation as a caress and as deeply pleasurable, like a bath. The melted state feels vulnerable, and

⚘ EVEN BETTER THAN A HOT FUDGE SUNDAE

When Jennifer was sixteen, her mother gave her a copy of *Autobiography of a Yogi* by Paramahansa Yogananda. He was one of the first swamis to bring meditation and yoga to the West, and his book has inspired millions of Americans (including Lorin and me). Jennifer loved his stories and began to meditate in a way that he describes, focusing on her "third eye" and filling it with blue light. Doing this made her happy in the midst of her teenage tribulations, and she continued this meditation for years. But at some point Jennifer realized that she felt removed and spaced out. When she had a child and needed to be more grounded, she stopped meditating.

In her sessions Jennifer, now thirty-five, expressed difficulty with boundaries and taking time for herself. As we explored these themes, she discovered that her usual way of paying attention was to be above and outside of her body in a hypervigilant surveillance mode—what I call "periscope attention." She described it as "watching my six, as if I'm in a fighter plane." (The military term "six," for six o'clock, refers to being aware of what is coming up behind you when you fear an attack.)

Jennifer found relief in learning to focus on concrete body sensations: the way her body rested on the pillow, the texture of the carpet, the movement of her breath, the sense of her muscles and skin, her awareness of the room. These sensory cues became ways to be herself and to establish a ground in pleasure. After experimenting with this focus for a week or two, Jennifer took a yoga class and noticed, "I was much more in my body. I had more awareness, and my mind was quieter than it usually is."

Jennifer was in a period of intense transition. "I'm scared, upside-down, topsy-turvy overall. I've set a bomb off in my life; I've upset the apple cart. I'm not doing things the way I used to, but I don't really have my hands on what that means. Meditation is very helpful in this transition. It is bringing me back. That's where my safety is; it's creating safety for me. I'm learning not to make so much effort. Meditation is the thing that's helping me go forward, and it feels really good. I enjoy my meditations so much and look forward to them with excitement. It's even better than a hot fudge sundae!"

you may wonder whether there are rules that you're breaking. You may even invent some. The very feeling that you are violating taboos is a sign of success; it means that you are going deep. It is a challenge to face this feeling, and you need to find ways to support yourself. So surrender to your own experience. Do not surrender to abstract ideas, techniques, or gurus. Get this point right away so that you don't bore yourself to death. Many women are afraid to really feel their sensuousness, or do not know how to, so their meditation becomes a very narrow experience. There is no hidden bonus to limiting yourself; you will simply not want to meditate.

You may as well construct your meditation practice out of what you love and enjoy, because then it is easier to pay attention and you *want* to meditate. One of the great secrets is how much fun meditation is. It

This technique fosters the state of deep relaxation. Consider it preparation for other meditations. Take a bath, as hot as you can comfortably stand, for up to half an hour. To help relax your muscles more, you can add a cup of Epsom salts. Use your favorite bubble bath or essential oils to delight your sense of smell, and light a candle if you'd like. Luxuriate in the satiny texture of the water and the penetrating heat. Have a glass of water nearby to quench your thirst.

Carefully get out of the tub. Wrap up in a sheet and lie down, covering yourself so that you do not get chilled. In that dilated state, get used to deep relaxation. Your muscles may feel like noodles, and you will probably sweat (very cleansing!). In that extremely relaxed state, let yourself drift and explore the sensations of letting go. Give

can even feel deliciously naughty. Once you know how, you may find that it is something you crave and even prefer over your "vices." Imagine how luxurious that is!

If you follow your own instincts, letting your own experience be the guide, you will discover secret pathways and secret pleasures. Each meditator, whether a teacher or a student, has found little joys about meditation, and tiny ways to observe, that no one else has discovered. If you were in a garden with a cat, a dog, a child, a gardener, an artist, and an entomologist, each one would show you a completely different world of delight, because each one enjoys a special aspect of the garden and explores it in a particular way. We've been listening to our students for thirty years and are always learning new things. Find your way— your unique, sensual, and womanly way.

EXPLORATIONS

- What are your favorite sights, colors, sounds, smells, tastes, sensations, and musical experiences? What makes you swoon?

- What gives you joy? What do you love?

- When have you felt most relaxed in yourself?

- When have you had a sense of satisfaction, such as the feeling many people have after a job well done?

- Take a moment to consider some everyday pleasure you indulge in occasionally. What daily activity gives you a secret pleasure? It could be putting on makeup or going to the store. Caressing the velvet of an evening dress. Having a good cry. Making a connection, a deal, a plan. Creating order in your home. Creating peace. Cooking for friends. Setting the table. Arranging flowers. Taking a bubble bath by candlelight, or a long hot shower.

- Throughout your day take any sense and "pleasure" it, then savor the aftereffects. We do this instinctively: smelling a fragrance and enjoying the lingering scent; caressing your body with lotion; melting ice cream slowly in your mouth. After stimulating that sense, let go and feel what happens. Notice how the sensation disappearing is just as pleasurable as the sensation itself. We don't always want the full dose, we want to rest and luxuriate in the subtleties. When you pay attention this way, how does your experience change? Jot down some notes about your discoveries.

> yourself at least ten minutes. Afterward you may want to take a cool shower and then apply a fragrant lotion all over your skin.

❧ SKILL CIRCLE #1:
HOW TO MEDITATE WITH THE PLEASURE OF THE BREATH

Breath is a classic focus for meditation, for several reasons. For one thing, what could be handier? Breath is sensuous, rhythmic, and always with us, as long as we are alive. Also, breath is a gift to us from the larger world; it comes inside our body, into our lungs, into our blood, then into every cell. Breath is an intimate exchange with the entire cosmos in which we live and move and have our being. In paying attention to a breath, we perceive all this directly. Breath is intrinsically full of grace.

There are hundreds of ways to pay attention to breath. You can be aware of its rhythm, of how it expands and contracts, of how it weaves from outside of the body to being drawn inside. You can visualize the breath, being aware of the tip of your nose, the quiet sounds of your breathing, the silky feeling in your throat, the pause at the end of the inhalation, and so on. You can focus through your sense of touch, movement, hearing, smell, or vision. You can use breath to withdraw from the world or to engage with it.

When you meditate with the breath, allow your eyes to be open or closed—whatever happens spontaneously. You will learn to rest in the presence of breath, and your eyes will tend to close by themselves, but don't force them shut. If you take this gentle approach, even the simple act of closing the eyes can feel exquisite.

Your thoughts will drift off and then return to your focus. This is natural. Just keep coming back to your chosen pleasure. And remember that you can sit anywhere and in any position that is comfortable.

Over time you will develop more and more sensory awareness of what breath is. As you do so, it will become more and more engaging. Eliminate the phrase "trying to concentrate on my breath" from your vocabulary, and replace it with "I am developing an interest in breath."

Use your senses to greet each inhalation. As you become more aware of breath, extraordinary realms of sensation open up.

Smell You can enhance your sense of smell by exploring the particular nuances of your favorite scent—a flower, essential oil, or ripe fruit—and the sensations of breathing it in. Then, as if appreciating an intoxicating fragrance, inhale slowly and savor the breath. Even if there is nothing actually in the air to be smelled, putting your attention in your nose as you breathe awakens the sense of smell.

Motion Be aware of the movement of your breath as it enters through your nostrils, streams down your throat, and expands your lungs, diaphragm, and belly. Notice the pause at the end of the inbreath, where it turns somehow to flow out, and then pay attention to the feelings that go with the exhalation. Observe what happens at the end of the outbreath: you are empty of air, and then the whole cycle begins again. Feel your natural breathing rhythm. Then play with the tempo, speeding up or stretching out the inhalation, then exhaling more slowly or more quickly. You may love the inhalation more than the exhalation, or vice versa, or you may love the place at the end of an inhalation where the breath turns. Notice these preferences and explore them.

Touch Enjoy the caress of the air as it flows through the nose or mouth, brushes the back of your throat, and enters your lungs. Feel the touch of the breath stretching you inside like a gentle massage. Where do you feel it? Breathe out through your lips or nostrils onto the skin of your arm and delight in how it tickles the little hairs. Sense the moisture or dryness as you inhale as well as the moisture of your exhalation.

Temperature The outside air and your body are often different temperatures. As you draw in the breath and expel it again, notice the cues that inform you of its coolness or warmth.

Vision If you love color, you could have a swatch of that color before you and open your eyes to look at it from time to time. Breathe in the quality of that color. Or imagine your breath as a colorful stream that swirls inside you and then flows out into the space around you. Play with the designs made by the pathway of breath.

Hearing If you crave music, you could play music for the first five minutes of a breath meditation, then sit in the silence for another five minutes. The rhythm and harmony of the music can influence your experience of breathing in many ways. Consider your breath itself as music; let it become audible in some way. Hear the passage of air through your nose or mouth and play with the sound—hiss, blow, or pant. Then try keeping your mouth closed and hear the sound coming from your throat. Gently constrict the back of your throat to create a kind of whisper or rushing sound—like the breathing of someone sleeping, or the sound of waves coming to shore. This is called the "Ujayi breath" in yoga. Listening to the sound of your breath is a strong focus for meditative awareness.

Check out these statements for breath awareness:

"Now I am aware of smelling the breath."
"Now I am aware of the motion of the breath."
"Now I am aware of the touch of the breath."
"Now I am aware of the temperature of the breath."
"Now I am aware of seeing the breath."
"Now I am aware of hearing the breath."

❧ MEDITATIONS

The Sensuousness of Breath

The quality of attention in meditation is exquisitely delicate. In this meditation and all the others you explore, never force or be hard inside yourself. Always let your awareness be soft and undemanding, like flower petals on your skin.

Sit comfortably for several minutes and let your senses catch up with the present moment. Then bring your attention to your breath and ask, "What pleasure do I feel in breathing?" As elucidated in the skill circle, any of your senses—or several simultaneously—can enhance your awareness of breath. How luscious can you let it be? Maybe you enjoy the relaxing ebb and flow of the breath, its silky texture, its fragrance, the internal massage of its wavelike movement, or the simple wonder of receiving this gift from life. Imbue the breath with any texture or quality you crave.

Breathe with awareness for ten minutes or so. You will drift off into thoughts or feelings about your life; this is a normal and healthy process of integration. When you notice yourself drifting, don't try to block out those thoughts. Just keep coming back to the sensuousness of breath when you can so that your whole being can dilate in pleasure and be nourished.

Breath meditations can be wonderful outside in nature, especially with a breeze or a wind blowing on the skin. Experiment. Each day you will discover something new and delicious about breathing.

Basking in Your Womanhood

Though we share the common state of being female, how each of us experiences womanhood is very individual. Bask in your own particularly female atmosphere. Celebrate your feminine form—breasts, hips, vulva—your unique incarnation of woman. What is it like to endorse yourself as woman? Steep yourself in that awareness and appreciate it thoroughly. Notice how balancing this "yes" feels. Stay with it for ten minutes, then gradually open your eyes. Take several more luxurious minutes to integrate the internal yes with the sense of yourself in the external world. Then when you're ready, go out and enjoy!

Music to Your Ears

When you're in the mood to be bathed in sound, it is wonderful to meditate with music (one of my absolute favorites). What kind of music do you crave right now? What matches how you feel today? Do you want something gentle and nurturing? Passionate and percussive? Classical, New Age, rhythm and blues? Instrumental or a song?

Turn the music on and sit comfortably where your spine can be vertical. Let your body be relaxed. There are two ways to meditate with music, and you will probably alternate between them. Each satisfies a different phase of meditation, so just go with your flow. There is no wrong way to do this!

One mode is to give the music your total attention. Listen with your entire body as if you have ears all over. Hear its mixture of melody and rhythm. Sense the motion in your body; sway gently or even hum or sing along. Completely give over to the feeling that the music evokes.

The second mode is to let the music be a supportive background atmosphere, more like an ocean of sound that surrounds you as you breathe. Choose a quieter, "meditative" soundscape that does not impose forcefully on the atmosphere. (A wealth of such music is available; see the recommendations at the end of the book.) Enjoy the pleasure of immersion in this atmosphere; let yourself be carried by the sound. You can let your head move subtly as you drift.

Music can be like food for your inner being. When you pay attention this way, your whole body absorbs the nourishment. You may feel the vibrations of sound like a loving touch on your skin, or you may find that you can drink the music in with your breath, like water for a thirsty soul. Sometimes I want the music to penetrate my body, so I turn up the volume and imagine it sinking into my bones, my belly, or my heart.

After five or ten minutes of listening, turn down the volume and for the next five minutes notice the aftereffects of the music: the rhythms you continue to feel, any emotions it stirs up, or subtle reverberations in the silence.

Mmmm Meditation

Now you get to be your own music and indulge thoroughly in the sense of delight. Play with the sound *mmmm,* starting with a low hum and then exploring and letting the rhythm, pitch, or volume change any way you wish. Notice how the hum resonates through your head, your chest, your entire body. Improvise. Hum the pleasure into every cell, all the way to your bones. Vibrate with bliss! When you feel finished, let the hum subside and take several minutes to savor the aftereffects. You can do more than one round of sound and silent sensing, entering each time into even deeper enjoyment.

≈ GOING FURTHER

Favorite Sin Meditation

Embrace a secret pleasure or vice as a meditation. This will give you some clues to your most cherished sensory pathways. When we are indulging in one of our favorite pleasures, our senses open up to delight in the way the world smells or tastes or looks. The more your meditation is formatted according to these pathways of pleasure, the more meditating fulfills you and ultimately preempts your bad habits. You can mine your vices for the healthful pleasures hidden within them.

What is your favorite "sin"? Making judgments about what constitutes a vice is so subjective—only you can determine what that is for you. You'll get no moralizing from us! Your vice may be something that gives you a certain feeling of luxury, a feeling that life is good, that you're really cool, hot, rebellious, sexy, or naughty. Though acting out your vice—for example, smoking, drinking, having too much coffee or food, spending a lot of money shopping—may be inadvisable, you can harvest the original pleasure and freedom behind it. It can even be something innocuous that nevertheless holds mischievous delight for you. Flirting, reading romance novels, or watching TV can all qualify. For example, my body can no longer tolerate my old vices, like drinking coffee or too much wine; the aftermath just isn't worth it. So I now get a lot of mileage out of my morning black tea. I used to think tea was "bad" (because of the caffeine) and would drink it anyway with gleeful indulgence. Even though tea has recently made it onto the list of healthful substances because of its antioxidants and other anticancer elements, I still cherish it as if I'm breaking a rule.

Bring the secret pleasure of your vice into meditation. Breathe with the delight and freedom the vice creates. Let that pleasure tickle your inner senses just as if you were acting out. For one minute sit with your eyes open and settle into the sofa or chair. Then think of your favorite sin for half a minute. Imagine how you would feel if you were savoring it now. How are your senses awakened? Let your mind drift and daydream for another half-minute. Then let your attention flow back and forth between re-creating that pleasure and drifting for another five minutes—or as long as you want to indulge.

The Secret Smile

This smile radiates through the three octaves of head, heart, and belly. Sit comfortably so that the three smiles are aligned. Each of these areas is a major center of energy, and it is especially important for women to know how to let each area relax and soften into openness. Give yourself a gentle face massage before you begin. (See "Stretch It Out" in "Secret #12: Live It Up.") Close your eyes and enjoy.

Settle in for several minutes and invite pleasure and relaxation.

Then bring your awareness to your forehead and wiggle your eyebrows gently to release the area. Imagine a smile that begins at the center of your brow and curls with ease up and out across your forehead. Feel how it spreads and smoothes any furrows away. Notice how just the suggestion of a smile evokes serenity and inner beauty. Enjoy these feelings. This is also the area of the "third eye," so don't be surprised if you see more light. (Bonus: this meditation can take years off your face.)

Now bring your awareness into your chest. Feel the movement of your ribs as you breathe. As you inhale, your chest stretches inside, gently expanding into more fullness. As you exhale, your chest softens. Imagine a huge smile that starts at the center of your chest and spreads up under your breasts, cradling and lifting your heart. Breathe in with comfort and joy.

Finally, draw your attention down inside your lower belly, beneath your navel and above the pubic bone. Rest your attention within the belly center for a moment. Imagine a curve at each side spreading upward into your hipbones, like a very private smile. Let your breath come to meet that area and infuse it with warmth.

These three smiles are like upturned crescents. Let them spread wide. Welcome whatever sensations, feelings, or images arise. For example, the upper curve may shine beyond your head, a silver crescent moon that crowns your hair like the mystic headdress of a high priestess. The heart smile may be a radiant golden light that glows warmly through your chest. The lower smile may be a vibrant molten red that melts and opens your hips. Your inner smiles may be Julia Roberts bright or enigmatic like Mona Lisa's, or they may be more like grins—a little sassy or sly.

Take your time to explore each smile, then all three together. The corners of your mouth will probably curve upward irresistibly; they'll want to play too. When you're ready, slowly open your eyes and relish the afterglow. Make a gradual transition, taking this secret smile into your life.

❦ REFLECTIONS

- Which of these sensory meditations gives you the most pleasure? Of the variations on simple breath meditations, which do you enjoy the most?

- As you give yourself this time out and time in for pleasure, do you encounter an injunction against "selfishness"? Do you notice any unspoken rule, like a taboo, that comes up as you enter such sensuality? If not, celebrate! Take yourself to lunch. But if so, whose voice is that? Do you really believe it or need it anymore?

- What permission can you give yourself now to take even more delight in your sensory experience?

- Other suggestions for responsible and healthful pleasures: frequent sex within a loving relationship; laughter; walks; talks with close friends; creative activities such as music, dance, and writing; meaningful work. Is there an area you would like to develop more?

- Remember this principle: pleasure, not work. Think of your focus on pleasure as a loving commitment to yourself. The techniques are not about "making something happen." (See "Secret #4: Be Tender with Yourself.") If pleasure seems foreign or hard to find, do mini-pleasures throughout the day. Pause in the middle of any activity that you enjoy. Just stop and drop into the moment to appreciate it. Let your awareness soak up all the pleasurable impressions. When you bring your attention to the sensations and perceptions in this special way, even for a minute, your whole being is suffused with life-affirming joy.

- You can start with one of these meditations and stay with it for a week or more. It will have much to teach you. You'll find that your sensory awareness in everyday activities is greatly enhanced and the world seems more alive.

🐾 SECRET #2
HONOR YOUR INSTINCTS

Slowly drifting awake . . .
Eyes flicker open, close again.
Body deliciously heavy with dreams . . .
A silky breeze seeps in through the window . . . the glint of dawn.
Softness of flannel sheets and squishy pillows,
The perfect weight of the covers . . . mmm, I am cuddled in coziness.
A sleepy smile pervades me:
Comfort—at home, on this bed, on this Earth.
Sweet moment, this . . .

I slip out of the nest to steal the precious solitude . . .
In the living room I re-create the cozy sweetness.
A fuzzy shawl wrapped around me like my own fur,
I sit and breathe the silence in.
I drink the breath like an elixir—oxygenated nectar refined
From the exhalation of trees and flowers and oceans wide . . .
What I breathe out in turn becomes their food . . .
Animal and plant in an eternal exchange—utterly interdependent.
Each atom of oxygen is immortal,
Combining and releasing through living forms around our planet,
Transformed but never changed.
I take my place in this seamless circulation,
Woven within the intricate interconnectedness of all life.

Sun rises, birds trill . . . the world is waking up.
My animal eyes open to the day, ears casually alert.
Saturated with pleasure, I slowly stand and stalk through the hall,

Ready for the familiar newness as the adventure begins again:
Human creatures discovering what it means to be alive.

❧ ❧ ❧

THE WISE MOTIONS OF LIFE

As women, we know that we are inextricably part of Nature—we smell, taste, hear, and breathe Her wisdom every day. When we recognize ourselves as creatures on this earth, the texture of life is both enriched and simplified. Metaphors reveal our inner nature and are not a far stretch from the literal. We are human beasts; we are walking trees; we are the soil that gives birth to new life. This awareness makes our needs immediate and clear. What does the creature self need to thrive? Tend to your inner nature, honor it in the movement of your life, and let meditation support this self-care.

To get the most out of meditation, expand on the prevailing limited views. There are two, one modern and one ancient. The newest, a by-product of scientific research, confirms that meditation is good for your health. This view sees meditation as a daily maintenance tool, a monotonous and mechanical routine like brushing your teeth; you hate to do it, but you figure you must. The other, older view is that meditation is arcane and elite, a complicated method for transcending earthly life. In both cases meditation is considered a man-made technology, like a new, improved toothbrush or a spaceship for interstellar travel. Although there is something to be said for each of these approaches, we want to call your attention to a simpler and more stunning paradigm.

Meditation is instinctive. It is natural. Your body already knows how to meditate—the ability is built in. Meditation is an aspect of the body's innate survival strategy, and it is good for healing, balancing, adapting to the environment, resting, recharging, renewing, and creating greater alertness. The body loves meditation and takes to it like a duck to water.

The techniques of meditation arise from the body itself. People fall into meditative states naturally and spontaneously for a moment here, a moment there. You already know times when you border on meditation or slip through into a meditative state: listening to music, watching a sunset, lying in bed after lovemaking. As you wake from sleep, and as you fall into sleep, there may be moments when you are very restful and yet awake inside. In meditation you learn to extend such moments of "restful alertness." What we are calling a technique is when you give in to this process for half an hour and let it carry you deep within.

Sometimes you are led into sublime realms that feel deliciously delicate. At other times you feel earthy, primitive, wild, and sexy. Learning to tolerate the coexistence of these opposites is one of the basic skills of meditation. The old stereotype of meditation is that it is rarefied, ethereal, abstract, and otherworldly; you "leave your body" and float around in the ethers. It is often implied in spiritual circles, or even overtly stated, that you are supposed to overcome your primitive urges and disown your instincts. Because people are used to thinking of the instincts as lowly, dangerous, and confusing, they try to control and transcend them. This one-sided stance is myopic, impoverished, and fragmenting. Such a limited view is based on a profound misunderstanding of spirituality. If you try to conquer your instincts, you will only succeed in being at war with your inner nature.

A healthy approach to spirituality embraces the full spectrum of human experience. You do not deny anything. Meditation is a vessel of awareness, and you bring your entire being into it. You welcome every impulse, every emotion, and every desire. When you pay attention to your inner life without prejudice, you begin to appreciate all these impulses as part of your body's innate intelligence. The instincts are sacred. They are the wise motions of life that impel us to survive, breathe, feed ourselves, rest when we are tired, heal, seek out friends, and join with mates. These natural movements are exquisite and precious. Engaging with the wondrous process of life renewing and sustaining itself on every level is a foundation of meditative practice.

When we honor our instincts, they put us in touch with our human creaturehood and with what we require to be healthy animals. When you embrace your instincts consciously, each one gives you a gift and enriches your life. As you meditate, you bring awareness to these movements that are usually subliminal. You give them all permission to be alive and shimmering in your being so that they can be integrated. Having lively access to your instincts gives you a robust vitality, so learn to befriend them all.

As the human brain has evolved, earlier development has not been abandoned, but built upon. Like evolution, meditation is an inclusive process. We actually have three brains, and each speaks to us with its instinctual wisdom. The most basic is called the reptilian brain, which includes the spinal cord and the brain stem. The reptilian brain clues us in to our primitive needs for safety, survival, and territoriality as well as the human need for order, regularity, and routine. Then there is the mammalian or limbic brain, and surrounding it is the cerebral cortex. The limbic system is the "seat" of the emotions; it connects us to our social needs, including our desire to bond and communicate with each other. The third, higher brain includes the neocortex and gives us consciousness—the ability to reason and to understand ourselves. As human animals, we need all three levels of knowing; we are not fully human unless all of these brains are functioning in synchrony. We see meditation as an essential action taken by the brain to tune itself up and strengthen the communication between all its parts.

Hunches, gut instincts, and intuition are forms of instinctive knowing. When the three parts of the brain are working together and all the instincts are flowing, we get revealing sensations. We call our responses to the outer world "gut instincts." When the senses track the inner world, we call it intuition. The fact that women process information with both the right and left hemispheres of the brain may account for our enhanced intuitive capacity.

With the development of the neocortex, humans became capable of self-reflection and acquired the ability to ponder the intricacies of the universe. It may even be that we now have an instinct to create meaning. Humans are able to perceive connections between different levels of experience and generate mythological significance. We love to learn and communicate through symbols, stories, music, science, and art. This human ability to create significance no doubt has evolutionary purpose. It is a scientific fact that having a sense of meaning is a prime factor for optimum physical and psychological health. Even such elegant responses as awe and wonder can be seen as part of our instinct to be oriented to the environment. Placing yourself within the "larger picture"—however ineffable that may seem—provides not only relief from existential isolation but a deep source of nourishment. Wonder is brain food. When we gaze at the stars, for example, we feel small, humbled within such vastness, but in touch with the mystery of our place within the whole. This experience points to a paradox about meditation: it is both primitive and refined.

Awe, gratitude, sorrow, longing, humor, and joy are all instinctive responses and can evoke spontaneous states of meditative awareness. People naturally pause in them—Ah!—but only for a breath or two. The

❧ NATURAL WONDER MEDITATION

You can build a meditation based on ways you naturally experience wonder and joy. Do this anywhere, anytime.

Facing a dawn, a mountain range, or the stars on a clear night, a sensation of wonder sometimes overtakes us. The wonder emerges from our core, from the deepest parts of our brain. It is a wordless recognition, but if you could put the feeling into words, they might be: *I exist as a very small part of this large and magnificent world.* Everyone knows this experience; it happens spontaneously given the right conditions, and it is an instant enlightenment. In that moment filled with wonder and awe you are enlightened.

Seek out these experiences in the outer world and expand your repertoire. In meditation you can also call up the memory and relive the times when you have been in natural wonder. The more you practice this, the better you get at the recall. In reliving such an experience, you can push the instant replay button and go over and over your favorite parts. This is not just an imagination exercise; it nourishes all of the senses. This prepares your nervous system to appreciate beauty and makes you better able to stop and receive the gift of these experiences when they come your way.

Call to mind one such moment and take a few breaths as if you were there right now. What are the particular sensations you feel in your body as you contemplate this aspect of life that fills you with wonder? Let your attention wander through your senses. What do you hear? What do you smell? What is the quality of light? What are you feeling in your belly, on your skin, in your heart?

List in a journal the times when you have experienced natural wonder. Then each day spend one or two minutes savoring those experiences. You will notice over time that you are subtly changed by this. You may find that you are more grateful to be alive.

secret is to stay there in the intensity and let it transform you. That is the secret of meditation: allowing life itself to inform, reform, and transform your sense of yourself and the world.

Be Natural with Yourself

Meditation happens spontaneously when you have the right conditions and you allow the natural process to unfold. You don't have to force anything. The body, in its wisdom, seizes the opportunity to heal and balance if you give it half a chance. Meditation is that half a chance.

❧❧ THE INSTINCTS IN THE OUTER WORLD

Everyday life is structured around the instincts:

- *Resting:* sleeping and dreaming
- *Feeding:* nourishing yourself and your family and pets
- *Grooming:* bathing and getting dressed, doing your hair, picking the nits out of your children's fur
- *Gathering:* foraging by going to the store or the garden and bringing food home
- *Hunting:* searching for what you need in the environment, shopping for the best buys, going for what you want in the world
- *Exploring:* looking and sniffing around to discover what interests you, going on adventures, expanding your horizons
- *Homing:* using navigational skills to find your way home when you have been out exploring
- *Nesting:* building a home and tending to it, decorating, cleaning, being cozy, snuggling in bed
- *Socializing:* talking on the phone, getting together with friends
- *Playing:* having fun, doing things for sheer enjoyment
- *Courting:* flirting, considering possible mates
- *Mating:* developing a love relationship, having sex
- *Procreating:* acting on the urge to bear children
- *Communicating:* expressing, singing out, saying what you know
- *Protecting:* looking after the self, the cubs, and the tribe
- *Establishing dominance:* competing in the workplace, finding your place in the pecking order

You have marked the time out and said to the nervous system, "You are free. I won't make you do anything else right now." The goal of all training is to be natural with yourself so that meditation does not feel like a technique at all but rather just a way of being with yourself. There is something wonderful and almost miraculous in how meditation works. If you do the simplest technique, in the easiest manner, you tend to enter a state of profound physical relaxation and regeneration.

When you are natural and unaffected with yourself, your experience changes continuously and your senses pulsate with novelty. You feel as

❧ THE INSTINCTS IN THE INNER WORLD

This is how the instincts work within you during meditation. Your experience will change every few minutes as you shift from one to the other.

- *Resting:* relaxing into a state of restfulness much deeper than sleep
- *Feeding:* taking nourishment from the silence, from the air, and letting your deepest cravings be fed
- *Grooming:* feeling a gentle massage of your nerves, skin, and senses
- *Gathering:* picking valuable things from here and there in the universe and holding them to yourself
- *Hunting:* moving through your inner world on a trail toward what you seek
- *Exploring:* strolling along inside yourself just for the adventure and to expand your horizons
- *Homing:* finding your way to the places inside yourself where you feel most at home
- *Nesting:* being at home in yourself and doing things to maintain the nest, feathering it, making your inner world stronger and more beautiful
- *Socializing:* hanging out with all your inner voices and attributes, listening to the conversations between different parts of your brain and body
- *Playing:* meditating for the sheer enjoyment of it
- *Courting:* exploring the possibility of making a union with some part of yourself you have not owned yet
- *Mating:* forming a deep bond with your inner self and letting your body be penetrated by love
- *Procreating:* nurturing within your body the new life impulses growing there, the new sense of self, carrying that sense of self to term
- *Communicating:* praying and saying what it is you want in meditation
- *Protecting:* using meditation to strengthen your sense of boundaries and enhance your ability to maintain them
- *Establishing dominance:* working out which parts of yourself will take priority at any given moment: the child, the sexual woman, the worker, the mother, the ancient crone

though the knowledge of how to meditate is your own, that this wisdom comes from inside you.

Many people who have studied the Eastern wisdom have been overcome by its dazzling riches and have come to feel that the knowledge resides outside themselves. They become dependent on external authorities and then are infected not only with the ancient wisdom but with many ancient superstitions as well. Many of our friends who walk Asian paths are still not at home in their own skins and bodies, even after twenty or thirty years of meditation. They have to call India to get permission to break their vegetarian diet and eat some fish.

The wisdom of India and Tibet is like a mountain range composed of jewels of all sizes, enchanting to behold by sunlight or moon. The wisdom of the instincts resides at ground level and is like dirt and water, soil and seeds, green plants and your own little garden. It is about living things, not jewels. The instincts are what life does; they are right here, pulsating in every breath and every beat of the heart. This is a humbler approach, but one that leads each of us to our inner life in our own native way. When you are natural with yourself, you always know how to enter the type of meditation that you need in the moment.

Not a Separate World

You can see from the lists of outer and inner instincts that meditation is not separate from life in any way, nor is it guided by a separate set of impulses. The same instincts that guide you in daily life also guide you in meditation. In addition to the basic impulses of eating and sleeping, you have instincts to learn, explore your environment, create a home, protect your loved ones, make alliances with others, communicate, and play. Each of these is a vital part of being human and actively guides you in every moment of every meditation. All of the instincts come into play when you meditate, and a technique is a way of cooperating with them.

For example, breath is a much-loved focus for meditation. And what is breath? It is the process of taking in life-giving substance from the air and assimilating it into your body. Air is our primary food—we consume hundreds of gallons of it a day. In twenty-four hours we breathe about twenty-two thousand times. To pay attention to this process is as basic and satisfying as eating a meal.

The urge to rest is another fundamental instinct. Every organism operates within a cycle of rest, regeneration, and action. You know how refreshed you can feel after a good night's sleep. During meditation the body often goes into a state of rest more profound than sleep. So the urge to meditate can be a response to the need for rest.

The urge to nest, to make a home for yourself and your family, is a deep craving. Meditation allows the human homing instinct to lead us into being at home in ourselves and in the universe.

The need for inner grooming is another strong impetus for meditating. Sometimes you feel as though your feathers are all ruffled or your fur is out of place; your inner hair is a mess. You have the wrong clothes on, or your aura is the wrong color. The quality of attending to yourself in meditation helps to put everything back in place.

There is something joyous about participating with any or all of the instincts. When the instincts work together, it is like a symphony. Spirituality can be looked at as the process of refining the instincts and bringing them into concert. Meditation is that time when the orchestra members come together to tune their instruments, warm up, synchronize, and prepare to perform.

Working with the instincts is always surprising, because there are so many layers of intelligence within each impulse. You pick up a clod of dirt from your garden, and upon closer examination you suddenly realize that each speck shimmers with multicolored light.

You do not need to impose the desire to meditate on yourself. The motivation is already there within your primitive desires. Life's timeless wisdom is pulsating within you as your deepest hankerings. Orient yourself to pleasure and let it be your guide. Get used to the idea that pleasure is instinctive. It is part of the great design of nature that rewards us when our basic needs are met: we take pleasure in drinking water when we are thirsty, in eating when we are hungry, in resting when we are tired. Approaching meditation as a healthy pleasure protects you in the long run from any negative side effects. You are activating your own self-correcting instincts.

HEALTHY BOUNDARIES

All organized systems and living things have auras around them, concentric spheres or living fields of force that filter energy from the universe to a level appropriate to their nature. The earth, for example, has many layers of atmosphere to filter sunlight to a level that sustains rather than kills life. A cell is surrounded by a membrane that selectively lets in nourishing elements and blocks out what is not.

Meditation is a place to cultivate consciously your own "atmosphere," your healthy aura. As a human being, you have a right to filter out what is harmful to you and to say yes to what helps you thrive. Healthy boundaries develop by exercising this choice. They take care of you. Being aware of your body is a way to sense your boundaries. Your skin is a membrane that distinguishes "you" from what is around you and helps you to feel the boundary of your personal space. Pause for a minute right now and sense your skin, your body, and where you are placed in your environment. How do you know what is you?

Choosing what goes into your body is a simple but powerful exercise of healthy boundaries. The orifices of your body are openings for choice: what you put in your mouth to eat, what you take into your eyes and ears, what enters the most private openings of the genitals. Knowing how you want to be touched is a boundary, and you can teach others how to touch you. In addition, the environments you expose yourself to, the people you choose to see, and what you do with your valuable time and energy determine your boundaries.

Healthy boundaries are the result of the interplay of all the instincts, not just one or two. It is one-sided and unbalanced to think of meditation as dissolving boundaries and merging with infinity. Meditation helps you know your boundaries and preferences, not erase them. Only when you know your boundaries is the expanded perception of no-boundaries, nonseparation, and oneness that also comes with meditation a life-serving, integrated state. Many women on a spiritual path miss this important point.

While you are meditating, a certain percentage of your time is taken up reviewing any "boundary invasions" you have experienced—times when you said yes but you felt no, or when you disrespected your own internal rhythms. In every evening's meditation the events of the day come to mind to be felt, and usually there is something about boundaries. If you have been too fierce during the day, bristling at every request, then you may find yourself moving in the direction of compassion, seeing the other person's point of view. But if you have been too gentle, too accommodating, then your meditation may lead you into seeing the wisdom of saying no. This is why it can be harmful to try to impose "virtues" such as compassion on yourself. Unless you are a really selfish person, cold and uncaring, you may not need to practice

ஃ **PILAR'S WATERFALL**

Pilar was born in Colombia into a large, close-knit family. Now thirty-seven, she runs a thriving business in Los Angeles. Pilar has a passionate heart, overflowing with love. She has also known great suffering, including the death of three brothers. "Even in my darkest moments, meditation helps me to celebrate life, to celebrate myself, so I don't take my pain and anger out on others. It teaches me how to receive as much as I give, and to find balance."

Pilar has created a little altar with a photo of herself as a child. "I need to stay close to my tears. Recognizing where I came from, my past, helps me to see my future. Meditating is like stepping down off a cement curb and onto the ground, sinking into the vastness of nature and my deepest feelings.

"I love to imagine myself in a forest by a stream, naked, with the wetness touching my body and the peaceful sound of a waterfall in the distance."

compassion consciously. In any case, the free flow of attention during meditation leads you into seeing and feeling balance.

Suppressing boundaries is a denial of the energy for self-preservation. A healthy immune system is a boundary—knowing what's "me" and what's "not me." Imbalance can be created in either direction: the rigid, walled-in boundary of "everything is not me," which is based in fear, or the flaccid lack of boundary, "everything is me, all is one," which is false surrender. Strong yet flexible boundaries give us integrity: the choice to say yes or no and mean it.

Saying yes when you mean no saps a great deal of psychic energy. This creates a lot of disturbance in your meditation: discomfort, emotional pain, and the noise of repetitive thoughts as you review the situation over and over. You can give yourself a break by learning to say no when you need to. The clarity and freedom of healthy boundaries can be yours.

AWAKEN YOUR ANIMAL POWER

In fairy tales, myths, and dreams, animals generally represent the connection to our bodies and instinctual knowing. They come as helpful allies, messengers, or guides to the seeker. Sometimes the dream animal that appears will be wounded or deformed—a sign that our relationship to the body requires healing, acceptance, and care. Always the creature gives us very specific clues to what is essential to our health, personal relationships, or creative expression and can reflect what we must do when our boundaries have become confused. They show us what energy must be accepted and embodied—from ferocious power to vulnerability or retreat. Reclaiming your creaturehood is a primary key to healthy freedom, joy, and comfort in your own skin.

Claire, a woman in her mid-fifties, journeyed to Los Angeles from New Zealand on a conscious and determined inner quest. Her occupation spanned from leading high-level career development seminars to clairvoyant dancing. Spiritually oriented and brightly positive, she had come to work with me to understand how to perform her dances and to open her body to subtler realms of energy and movement.

Claire's burning desire for truth made her rigorously honest. In her first session she admitted to constant pain in her sacrum and problems in her lower back that had plagued her "forever." We entered into a body meditation, which immediately revealed that something in there was snarling. She was astonished but willing to go with whatever showed up.

When I asked her to stand and explore the sensations, an image appeared to her—a tiger trapped in a cave. Courageously breaking life-long taboos on expressing anger, she became the tiger, pawing the ground and pacing in rage. Though letting vocal sound come out was still too terrifying to her, Claire nevertheless knew that the tiger was loose. Energy coursed from her pelvis through her legs and up through her spine. With it came tears of sadness—and relief.

The next morning Claire reported that for the first time in many years her back was free from pain (and it would remain so). Days later in her meditation the tiger was sitting outside the cave in the sun, happily licking its fur with a big pink tongue. Tending to her tiger self has become an ongoing way for Claire to stay true to her body and emotions. A year later she writes, "There is much awakening in my pelvis. I am becoming aware of vast resources of energy pulsing, surging, flowing, available. I feel beautiful, rich, golden, sensual, and vital."

Among the thousands of women we have worked with through body meditation and expressive movement, I cannot recall a single one who did not discover healing and liberation through her instinctive animal power.

EACH DAY IS DIFFERENT

When you follow your instincts, you have a marvelous sense of choice. Discovering how you want to meditate each day is a lot like going shopping. Think of it—shopping is a deep primordial instinct! Early woman knew when her tribe needed some variety in their diet and would go out and find the exact root or herb that provided those nutrients. You possess the same intuitive ability to select functions in your inner world: you forage or shop for your daily technique to find what satisfies your need that day. Here's how Lillian, an experienced meditator, puts it:

"Each day is different, so I dabble around and choose what meditation feels right for this moment. It's like multitasking, which women are so good at. Women need to have access to all their tools. I wear a tool kit on my hips, like the workmen and their leather belts with all those tools on them. Men seem to go through a change every six weeks; I've studied them and observed this. They go into their cave; they withdraw in different ways. But for women every single day is different, like the weather. There is not just one thing to do that suits my nature."

The inventiveness of women knows no bounds. Give yourself freedom to choose where you meditate, your style for the day, and even what you wear. Step into your wardrobe and play. Perhaps you have power clothes or jewelry, like amulets signaling the tone you want to create. Some days you may come out of the shower and want to put on your most beautiful silk; other days you may want to be butt naked, or adorned with only a necklace and rings. If you feel like Artemis (or Diana), you may need to be outdoors for a walking meditation, or sitting on a rock in the woods, or lying in the grass. If you've been out in the garden, the most pleasurable thing may be to stay there and meditate covered with mud. If you yearn to surrender in ecstasy, play music that inspires you, dance, or chant. Solitude and darkness may be what you crave, so you could meditate in the containment of a closet to feel safe. Or if a cozy nest seems most appealing, you could snuggle under the covers in bed. Each of these tones fulfills one of your instincts, and to give it gratification is pure delight.

Try meditating after exercise, in the afterglow of sex, or when you're filled with the emotional richness from a good movie. I've been known to watch tapes of the hilarious improvisations on the TV show *Whose Line Is It Anyway?* I laugh uproariously out loud (even when I'm by myself) and then meditate with the sense of humor still bubbling through me. Discover your weird and wonderful idiosyncrasies and revel in them brazenly.

A Mother's Nurturing Meditation

One day Lorin visited his sister Danielle to help her with her computer. She had a six-month-old baby at the time, and as soon as Lorin saw Dani, he said, "You look radiant, like you have meditated." Dani said, "No, I didn't meditate today." Persisting, Lorin kept asking, "When did you get up? What have you done all day?" Dani said, tiredly, "Well, I got up at three to feed the baby and sat in the living room nursing him. Then I sat there while he slept." With some further prodding, she admitted, "I sat there for quite a while—I was not sure whether I was awake or asleep. The whole world was quiet. The windows were open, and I could hear every sound, every whisper of the wind in the trees. I felt the whole neighborhood, and felt what a peaceful world I have brought this baby into. I would drift off and then return to awareness of holding this little love-bundle in my arms."

She was in mama-meditation, resting within herself and gathering her strength while also engaged in the activity of nurturing. This is an example of how something so basic and instinctive is also so sacred. Danielle was in the realm of the Goddess, feeling life flow into her, through her breasts and into her baby.

Even if you are not nursing, your meditation may at times feel as if you are holding yourself in your arms, loving and comforting yourself, a tired, discouraged woman who has just returned from a long day at work. As you rest within yourself you become aware of your inner strengths, the deep and powerful part of you that has unbounded love to give.

THE YOGA OF THE INSTINCTS

Approaching meditation as instinctive perception has an interesting effect in daily life—it lubricates the doors and gears, so you are not stuck in one limited mode of reacting to circumstances. Most of us realize after the fact how we could have dealt with a difficult situation. Given enough time, we develop twenty-twenty hindsight. It may take days, weeks, months, or years, but we get it eventually.

Meditation helps to shorten the learning curve. It creates more space, a gap between the stimulus and response, so that you become more flexible and can choose to respond as needed. Instead of realizing later what all your options were, you have more of a choice in the present moment. Time is collapsed; the future is brought forward into the present.

How this happens is no mystery. When you meditate every day, about half the time is spent in review of the day, and as you see the mental movies playing, you see how you could have responded better. This review almost always hurts: it's a litany of "ouch," "ah!," "ugh," and "oh, no!" The review happens only when you relax deeply, and as you do so something else happens: you learn to stay at ease while replaying the most tension-producing aspects of your daily life. In the situation under review you may not have been aware of all your choices, but in the ease and safety of meditation you can see them more clearly. This is not just "I coulda" or "I shoulda" thinking; the body is doing something really valuable. It is practicing more creative responses, and you will soon find yourself acting with greater range in your life.

When you cultivate the instincts in meditation and let yourself flow through them, you have more access to them in daily life. Your behavior is more resilient and adaptive. We all have our favored instinctual responses. In meditation, because it is about balance, your nervous system brings up the responses opposite to the ones you are comfortable with. You have been practicing letting yourself shift between resting and being alert, feeding and sensing boundaries, communing and confronting, and you end up quicker on the uptake in daily life. This happens so that you can get used to them and practice, in the safety of meditation, how to be with them. Because all your instincts are available to you, you get a richer sense of your options.

We call this "the Yoga of the Instincts" because it seems that the body flexes each of its instinctive responses in turn, like an athlete stretching every muscle in her body, going through pose after pose. In meditation the body often continues doing this until it strikes just the right balance or combination of instincts. The nervous system and body are trying on modes of approach, feeling them all out—defending, communicating, standing your ground, giving ground, exploring new ground, socializing, playing. There are infinite gradations to each possible response, and sometimes the body seems to want to ratchet through them all to find the optimum response. In the beginning this process can feel exceptionally bothersome and tedious.

Say the tense situation was with a coworker: you thought you were attacked, so you responded with a counterattack and told her off. But later, when you are at ease, watching the "movie" play again, you see everything with X-ray eyes. As you are sitting there, relaxed, your emotional body runs through the confrontation and tweaks your emotional dials in every conceivable direction. The replay may start with even more anger, then less, then apologies, then communication from the heart, then avoidance, then, surprisingly, playfulness. You may start laughing. The next day at work you have a lot of choices. And if you choose to make amends, you may not feel so serious—you may be laughing at yourself when you tell her the story of realizing you weren't being attacked. You find that you are not stuck in a fixed position, you are more open to hearing other points of view. Depending on how safe you feel in your meditation in general, the instinct yoga may be very surprising— you may find your body coming up with responses that have never occurred to you, that aren't even part of your habitual personality.

When situations come up, it's as if there is a silent "choice point," where you have a breath to pay attention to your gut feelings, your heart, your head, and to synthesize them all into one unified movement. It's easier to follow your impulses. The feeling is subtle; mostly you feel livelier. This all happens as a side effect of meditation. The world is a different place, a very different place, when you are relaxed and connected.

In emergencies you may find yourself being very clear. One day in a meditation group Lorin asked people what effect meditation was having on their daily life. They had all started three months before. Helen, a nineteen-year-old woman with a shy demeanor, spoke up. She had a part-time job in a manufacturing facility in Irvine, California. She had been working there for two months and was still considered a low-status newcomer. One afternoon a worker was injured—Helen heard a shout, looked over, and saw people gathering around the wounded person. Helen stood there for a heartbeat, taking it in, then realized that no one else was doing anything—everyone was in shock. Even the managers were simply saying, "Oh, my God!" Helen caught a glimpse of someone on the floor bleeding and realized that every second counted. Without asking for permission, she raced to the phone, called an ambulance, and had already gotten through when someone yelled out, "Call an ambulance." She put down the phone, stood there for another

moment, then in her mind's eye saw a clear, maplike image of the build-
ings and the roads around it. She realized that the building they were in
was one of dozens of identical structures inside a mazelike complex,
and that the ambulance would probably have trouble finding them. So
without wasting a second to explain herself, she dashed out of the
building at a dead run, went to the gate, and ordered the guards to open
the gate and keep all cars out of the way. When the ambulance
approached, she flagged it down, jumped in, and guided it to the best
spot to park. Then she escorted the ambulance out of the complex again
to make sure it didn't get lost on the way out. Finally, she returned to
work and calmly resumed her duties.

Looking back on this experience, Helen said, "Before I started
meditating, I would never have acted so quickly. I was confident in
myself and did not hesitate to do what was needed." She was quite
startled with herself, because how she had acted did not fit her picture
of herself at all. In particular, she was surprised with the utter clarity
with which she issued orders to all these older people.

Acting instantly on instinct is very different from waiting even a few
seconds. In situations such as the one Helen found herself in, waiting
can cause different impulses to collide in your stomach, confusing you.
Helen experienced a series of impulses to communicate, instruct, and
navigate. No internal noise prevented her from acting. Nature wants us
to be as supple as cats, able to shift from total relaxation to maximum
alertness in a moment if needed, and then to shift to being at ease again.
Many of us, however, are a bit like the Tin Man—creaking when we
move in an unaccustomed way, needing to put oil in our joints and to
work them in all directions.

Instinct yoga happens spontaneously in meditation as long as you
trust the process. All yogas are refinements of natural actions. Hatha or
physical posture yoga is derived from stretching. Animals, dogs, cats,
and kids stretch spontaneously. Hatha yoga is an intensification of this
instinctive action—in a relaxed fashion you move through a set of
poses, taking each joint through its full range of motion, moving the
body through every angle it can move. Now consider what the equiva-
lent of that would be with the instincts: trying each one on, feeling it,
holding it for a minute, then moving to the next. Mantra yoga is an
amplification of our natural tendency to hum to ourselves and to have
tunes running through our heads. Lovers devise inventive positions for

❧ GOLDIE'S WAY

The actress Goldie Hawn has a particularly earthy way to meditate in stressful circumstances. "I'll literally excuse myself and sit on the toilet somewhere to clear my mind. Pulling the energy in and getting the rest out, the debris, is very important." How's that for an example of creative and instinctive adaptation?

"Women are the healers and the caretakers and the heart of the home. They are very powerful," Goldie continues. "Women run households, they raise children, they have to be very, very tough. And when that power gets into the conference room, sometimes it's scary. . . . Women must be real, and they must also be feminine. . . . I'm not afraid of my femininity, and I'm not afraid of my sexuality, it's not about conniving to get what I want. It's about being true to who I am and taking pride in it."

Goldie long ago incorporated meditation into her everyday life. She has created a special shrine in her home, decorated with crystals, prayer beads, and Buddhas. She calls it "a sanctuary to house my spirit."

sex and sometimes linger there in the deliciousness; tantric yoga takes this inventiveness and lingering to even greater heights.

This is how more instincts become available to you in real-life situations and how you become more versatile. As that happens, you are better able to respond to the larger, overall situation. You're not stuck in acting from an image of yourself. It is important to embrace consciously your instinctive versatility. As you change, you become less predictable and less compliant. Your boundaries become clearer. Some people may not like this—they are no longer able to manipulate you. During the day, as you notice your choices, honor them.

❧ EXPLORATIONS

- There are many instinctive moments in life that border on meditation and can serve as gateways to that state: sitting in your nest, just being with yourself; snuggling in bed; gazing at the horizon; taking a bath with candles; praying; tending your baby; that half a second of pure pleasure while inhaling the smell of food. Which such moments can you recall?

- When do you feel most natural, most comfortable with yourself?
- When do you naturally shift into relaxation mode?
- Remember some moments of wonder, awe, and joy: giving birth, or attending a birth; contemplating the night sky; waking up to a glorious sunny day and being happy to be alive.
- When have you followed your gut instincts? What did it feel like?
- What have you learned about saying yes to what your body wants and needs?
- How easily can you say no when necessary?
- In dreams and mythic imagery, animals are often helpful or they carry a message. Each creature—dolphin, tiger, horse, bear, wolf, weasel, elephant, mouse, bird, lizard, snake—brings a different quality. Which animals do you feel the most related to? Which have appeared in your dreams? On your own or (even more fun) in a group, explore making animal sounds: grunt, growl, whimper, purr. Get primitive!

❧ WARM-UP: WALKING IN NATURE

This is an exercise in sensory awareness as you move through the environment—a forest, park, beach, or your own backyard. Even in a city there must be some nature somewhere!

Walk at a leisurely pace and let all your senses become alert, as if you've just awakened to the world. Bring your attention to your eyes as they take in the colors, shapes, and movement of life around you. Bring your attention to your ears and focus on the subtle layers of sound. Breathe in the variety of smells.

Stop occasionally to savor these impressions. Become aware of how your feet snuggle into the ground and cherish that contact. Touch the bark of trees and run your fingers through the grass, weeds, or soil. Smell a flower or leaf. Lift a rock or pebble and feel its shape and heft. As you walk, explore the particular way your weight shifts between your feet. At some point pick up the pace and sense how powerfully your legs and hips propel you through space.

Notice your responses. What in this environment are you instinctively drawn to? Does anything repel or scare you? What new information do you receive about the natural world and your relationship to it?

&& SKILL CIRCLE #2:
HOW TO MEDITATE WITH THE INSTINCTS

The instincts are movements that your body knows how to make. Meditation allows you to tune in to the specific wisdom of each one. This instinctual knowing comes into play in how you choose your daily focus in meditation as well as in what goes on during the process. A meditation technique is a way of cooperating with one or more of these movements, allowing it to lead you into your inner world.

Over time get to know all of these instincts as they function in your meditation and in your daily life. The ones you leave out will cause you trouble. Power comes from riding the instincts. As you honor each instinct, it guides and blesses you.

The more instincts you honor, the juicier and more productive your meditation will be. The instincts serve your meditation, and you can serve the instincts. The techniques of meditation occurred spontaneously to the sages of old; they happened instinctively. As you get the hang of this, your own techniques will occur to you.

Give yourself permission to enter any instinctive state at any moment, in response to your perceptions and inner callings. Being a healthy creature means being flexible enough to move in any direction at any time, to be responsive to whatever the situation calls for.

When you get stuck in meditation, it is often because you are denying or resisting one or more of the instincts by trying to cling to the ones you know. Let the diversity of instincts alert you to the richness of meditative experience. Be willing to be surprised by the unique way the instinctive tones alternate and interact each moment of your meditation. You will circulate through any number of these tones.

Minute Meditations with the Instincts

To get familiar with the instincts, take each one and meditate on it for one minute. Each day be with one, two, or three of them. Come up with your own one-word mantra for an instinct, such as "home," "nourishment," "shelter," "union," or "communion." Think its name and let the sound and quality it evokes permeate your entire being. This prepares the ground for the other meditative exercises you choose to do.

- *Homing:* Developing a sense of where home is within you. Being safe enough to relax and be yourself. "I am at home within myself. I am at home in the world. I am safe here."
- *Nesting:* Building an inner nest. Feathering it. "I am cozy in my inner world. I am free to adjust everything to suit my needs."
- *Resting:* "I am at rest in my inner sanctuary."
- *Grooming:* Bathing, putting yourself together inside, getting an internal massage. "I bathe in the air. I bathe in light. I bathe in silence."
- *Gathering:* In meditation you gather what you need today from your internal world. It can happen in an instant. You reach out into breath or sound or touch and gather in the energy substance you crave. "I gather what I need, all the energy and focus I will need today. I gather my thoughts and feelings."
- *Nurturing:* Taking in the nourishment that you have gathered. Learning how to be nurtured, finding when and how much you need. Knowing how to stop and digest your experience. "As I rest, I absorb the nourishment, I let it soak in and become part of me."
- *Protecting:* A sense of the integrity of your own space. Practically speaking, turning off the phone so you are not disturbed in meditation. Strengthening and claiming your boundaries. "I can protect myself. I am alert to my boundaries and can sense when they are invaded. I am surrounded by an aura of protection."
- *Hunting:* In hunting your senses are alert to your environment; you listen, you look, you smell. This instinct in meditation ferrets out the technique you need that day. It also lets your meditation strengthen you to create what you desire in your life. The flip side of hunting is hiding, or the sense of being hunted and the need for retreat. "All my senses are alert to my internal and external environment; I hear, see, smell, and feel in all directions. I can wait, being totally silent with my senses wide open. I can find the technique I need today."
- *Healing:* Regenerating. Licking your wounds. Meditation is a healing state in which your whole system can come into balance. "I am bathed in healing energy. I am in rapport with nature and the healing power of my own body. In the safety of meditation I acknowledge the hurts and let them be cleansed and dressed with soothing balm."

- *Exploring:* A sense of adventure, the desire for new experience, and the willingness to change. Utilizing your natural curiosity, you satisfy your desire to wonder and to wander with this instinct and let your mind expand. This ability is an aspect of adaptability. "I am on an adventure, open to new experience and willing to be changed by it. I am curious, full of wonder."

- *Playing:* Play is more than just the spontaneous activity of children. Play is creating space so life can move through you, free of a tight, serious tone. Play is the attitude of delight you take when you are involved in recreation. "I am in delight, and I playfully engage with my inner world."

- *Socializing:* Communion, socializing with all your parts, all your inner worlds. Reflecting on your outer relationships—a very natural female task. You get in touch with the love and longing in your heart. Preparing for outer socializing, like putting on your makeup and getting dressed for a special event. Getting ready to engage with the world. "I am in communion with all my inner voices and outer bonds. I am centered in the midst of my heart-connections."

- *Mating:* Mystical union, or internal union, the marriage of opposite parts of yourself. The willingness to open to love. Your natural eroticism and ability to surrender to the sensuous touch of life energy. In meditation inner mating gives birth to creative inspiration and lively impulses for expression in the world. "I am open to love within myself. I surrender to the delicious flow of energy in my body, and between body and soul."

The Spiritual Side of the Instincts

As you pay attention to any instinctive sensory tone, it engages and integrates with the others and refines itself as appropriate. You usually don't need to work consciously to refine an instinct; just allow it free play.

- *Exploring* turns into awe and wonder, research, wonder about creation, a wondrous relationship with God.

- *Mating* turns into an erotic, deeply pleasurable relationship with life, internal unions, and union with God.
- *Resting* turns into an ability to rest in God, to be completely at peace in the universe. Sometimes a nap is the most sacred meditation.
- *Nourishing,* taking food in, can be a deeply reverent and gracious activity. You are open to the bounty of the earth and the sea, as blessed by the sun's light, consciously accepting it into your body as a gift to renew and restore you. Eating can be a prayer: give us this day our daily bread.
- *Socializing,* joining with others in community, can transmute into a feeling of community in spirit.
- *Self-preservation* leads to doing things to live a healthier life, to make the world a better place for your children, to contribute something to the world that will be lasting.
- *Self-assertion* leads to inhabiting your individual life while also appreciating the differences in others. You gain the courage and determination to step out of the crowd and make your mark on the world.

We recommend not trying to modify or tone down any of your instincts. Get them to work together and balance each other, and let them continually evolve to new levels of integration.

The Skill of Playing

Cultivate a playful attitude. All mammals learn through play. Human beings crave variety and novelty, and meditation is like an adventure. During meditation we perceive something, some quality of breath or sound or light. Because we're in a safe situation and do not have to work for survival, the nervous system starts to play around with different ways of perceiving the same thing. Subjectively we may feel little more than quiet interest, but this state makes room for the improvisation that lets us see our lives anew. It's always surprising. Keeping an attitude of play helps you to accept the unpredictability and novelty of each moment in meditation.

❧ MEDITATIONS

The Elixir of Life

Let yourself settle in for a few minutes wherever you are—in your meditation spot or outdoors.

Step 1 Sit or lie down, letting your eyes open or close as you wish. Ponder this: How do you know in this moment that you are alive? What are the clues? Stay with this question for several minutes, exploring whatever you discover. Then when you're ready, gently proceed to . . .

Step 2 Now ponder this: In what ways are you well? What are the clues to your health in this moment? Notice any tendency to dwell on how you are not okay—a common habit of many women. Keep bringing your focus to the many ways in which you are actually well right now, however faint or tiny those impressions seem. Thrive in this awareness.

Step 3 Inhale deeply and slowly. Drink in the breath like precious nectar and receive its vital force. Recognize that the oxygen you take in is distilled from all the plants of land and sea. As you exhale, send your breath out as a gift back to nature. Imagine the great trees all over the world receiving your breath. Again and again breathe and savor this generous flow in and out. The simple circulation of the breath weaves you into the web of life on this planet, the home we all share. Take strength from that connection, your place in the fertile ecosystem of the earth.

The Movement of No

The ability to say no with clarity is a great pleasure. There is a paradox: no is always a yes to something else. This is the joy and freedom of healthy boundaries.

Step 1 Every woman could use ten different ways to say no. Practicing in meditation allows you to stay more relaxed when you need to exercise the no in life. Begin by standing. Inhale fully, drawing your hands in toward your body. As you exhale, say no and move your hands outward. Do this ten times, varying the tone of voice and quality of movement each time. Include in your thoughts any situation in which you need to establish a stronger boundary.

Step 2   Now pause and enjoy the effect of your movement. What sensations are you aware of in your body? How does your breath move? How do you experience yourself? If emotion comes, what does the feeling tell you?

Step 3   Remain standing, sit, or lie down to deepen into meditation with these impressions. Silently now, repeat the no a couple of times with your inner voice. Feel how the energy of the word clarifies your mind and body—your entire "atmosphere." Notice how relaxed you can remain. Then let go of the no and open to the yes. Breathe in with the power of choice.

The Earth Circuit

Since the human animal has evolved to an upright stance and a vertical spine, our bodies have a particular relationship to the electromagnetic field of the earth. A primary pathway of life force is up your back and down the front of your body in a continuous circuit—the "Earth Circuit."

Sit so that you can feel your spine tall and free, upright but not stiff. (If possible, sit directly on the ground—it's okay to support your back with a wall or tree and to let your legs stretch out.) Let your weight drop down through your hips and bring your awareness to the floor of the pelvis where you make contact with the ground, cushion, or chair.

Then, imagine that your "sit-bones" and tailbone reach downward like roots, deep into the earth. Feel or imagine them drawing energy into the base of your pelvis and up into your spine. Slowly follow the path upward through the center of your back. Take your time. Let your awareness slide up over the top of your head, then flow down your face through the front of your body to reconnect with the ground. Begin the cycle again. Ride the full circuit, the uninterrupted circulation up from the earth and back down. Enjoy the streaming of energy, noticing whether the speed wants to change in any way. Sense how the full circulation weaves your whole body together.

Explore the Earth Circuit for about ten minutes. Remember that it is natural to drift off occasionally; when you notice this happening, simply and gently return to the focus. At the end of your meditation, include a few minutes to come gradually to standing and continue to sense this flow. As your feet connect with the ground, they too are like roots that channel the life force through your legs. This is wonderfully energizing and balancing for your entire system.

&8 GOING FURTHER

Healing Meditation

This meditation is for whenever your life force is low and you are tired, depleted, or ill.

First establish your meditation nest. Curl up anywhere comfortable—in bed under the covers, on the sofa, or on cushions on the floor. Give over to the sensations of fatigue. Let your body fall into the ground, your muscles hanging heavy and relaxed. Feel the support from the broad and massive body of the earth beneath you.

Then become aware of the air all around and above you. Imagine that it is saturated with healing power. Know this as the benevolent loving atmosphere of Earth, the Great Mother's breath that surrounds and permeates us always whether we are aware of it or not. Rest in this healing presence; let yourself be bathed and nurtured by it. With each inhalation, gently draw from that nourishing atmosphere. Feel how each breath effortlessly carries that healing quality into your lungs, into each cell of your body, and into each secret place in your heart.

Creature Meditations

Totem Animal   This can be done sitting, standing, or moving around. You can explore in the privacy of your living room or in a public venue. (Nobody has to know what you're doing!) Practice this by yourself or in a group, and have fun. Ready?

Choose a creature as your power animal. Which one do you identify with or want to be more like? Meditate on becoming that creature. Use your imagination to enter its perceptual world. First, take a few minutes to settle in. Imagine you are in the animal's natural habitat and gradually begin to open your senses. Let your ears become alert. As this creature, how do you listen to what is around you? Let your eyes become its eyes. Open and close them at will. How do you see? Become aware of your nose; let your nostrils move slightly as you sniff the subtle scents on the wind. Do you have whiskers? How does your head move as you scan the environment? Bring your attention to your skin and imagine it as the fur or scales or feathers of your animal self. How does the skin make contact with the air, or water, or ground? How does it like to be touched? What about your feet and hands? Are they winged, finned, clawed, hoofed? Tense and release the big muscles of your thighs and buttocks. Are they haunches, powerful and mobilizing? How do they like to engage to propel you? Let yourself move in some way to get the feel of the whole body of this creature and how it inhabits its world.

What does this animal know? What does it want to teach you? What does it know about comfort? What is its particular sense of power? How would it react if sensing danger? Or a mate? Or its favorite food? What does it require to thrive? Let your own body absorb these qualities. Now or later, when you see other "humans," be curious about them as fellow creatures. What is your response to them?

Bask in Your Creaturehood   This is utterly easy and pleasurable. The technique can be done on its own or after one of the other meditations. In any comfortable position whatsoever, recognize yourself as creature—a human animal intrinsically part of the whole of nature. Bask in the ease, health, and power of that awareness. Let your body be relaxed and alert, enjoying the creature comfort within your own safe habitat. That's all! If thoughts about your daily concerns arise, accept them as how the human beast prepares to meet its environment. Then bring your attention back to the focus: the simple impressions of creaturehood.

❧ REFLECTIONS

- What is your relationship to nature?
- From exploring these meditations, what did you discover about your inner nature? Which instincts are most active in you or familiar to you already? Least familiar? Which are most comfortable? Uncomfortable?
- Which instinctual mode do you crave the most?
- When you meditate with your totem animal, how do your senses open up? Afterward, do you notice anything different in your relationship to the environment around you? How do you feel in your body? What is the gift of this animal friend?

- Imagine yourself in your ordinary world with your instincts awakened in this way. How do you feel inside now as you see yourself in daily life? Own the strength, vitality, alertness, and whatever other qualities you are aware of. Notice how the instincts inform you of your needs and how to get them met. Is there a particular issue you're dealing with where you could use more of this awareness?

- Draw or paint any impressions from these meditations. A specific image may come to mind, or your impressions may be expressed as abstract swirls, swashes, or lines. As you draw, let your hand choose the colors instinctively and move over your page with the qualities you feel inside. Then, after you finish, take a few minutes to meditate on the colors and forms you have created.

- As time goes on, keep track of your instincts and how they empower you in every area of your life.

❦ SECRET #3
CLAIM YOUR INNER AUTHORITY

Okay. This is a big day, challenging. I want to have all my ducks in a row.

What if people don't like what I say? What if they criticize, or worse, attack?

Uh-oh, I am way outside myself. Better come back.

Hurrumpf—giving my power away again. It just seeps right out like sap!

I'm going to settle in, meditate, and get myself together.

Containment and protection . . . that's what I need.

I place myself inside an imaginary sphere of energy—my sacred space.

I wrap my attention all around me, 360 degrees.

Here at the center I sit. . . . Hmm, it's as though I'm on a throne.

Yes, let's make it a stone throne, carved from ancient earth.

But I care not for dominion over others; it is sovereignty over myself that I demand.

No, not even demand—assume. I know this for inalienable truth.

No need to prove anything, to push or pull. Ah . . .

Amazing. The power floods back into my body,

Like a transfusion of my own blood.

This is my body. This is my life.

Oh. I see. . . . No one else can give me power.

And no one can take it away.

Nobody else knows what I should do or be.

Someday I will simply rest in this truth.

Someday all women will remember their sovereignty . . .

Now there's a prayer.

Deep inhalation: "My body, my breath, my life."

Each breath is permeated with pleasure and strength.

This is my atmosphere, unruffled and clear—
Full with my own essence, not owned by others' thoughts.
Deep exhalation . . . I am ready now.

🐎 🐎 🐎

YOUR GIFT

Life wants us. It wants all that we are.

The essence of meditation is to be centered in your inner authority, then come out in the world and act with power, integrity, and grace. It is not arrogant to claim your own authority. It is deeply responsible.

The process of becoming your full self is called individuation. To individuate is to grow beyond collective and conventional standards and to take responsibility for your own values. You are no longer a child, in a parental relationship with God or society, but fully inhabiting your own creative engagement with life.

To be truly yourself, to risk being different from your culture, family, or friends, can bring up anxiety and doubt. But your authenticity is in fact a gift back to your community. Each of us has a knowing that contributes to the whole. When you embody what you value and perceive, the fabric of connection between us all is enriched.

Authority and authenticity come from the same root that means "creator." Like the artist at the fringe of society or the shaman who dances at its outskirts, you may be one who receives a healing vision or speaks a truth that is desperately needed for the tribe. Our survival and development as a species depend on such communication, and now more than ever women's voices need to be heard.

SOVEREIGNTY OVER THE SELF

Every woman has somewhere within her a sense of her own authority, a sense of sovereignty. As women we know things through our bodies, emotions, and intuition—we call it female power, and that's just the way it is! When meditation validates this ability, a profound, healing integration takes place in body and soul.

Meditation can be a tremendous boon to women in coping with the outer world. When you meditate and honor your instincts, you tap into your inner knowing and become more confident. Afterward you often are aware of both the big things and the little things that want to change in your life. With your inner clarity, decisions seem to make themselves. This is a natural and spontaneous by-product of meditative awareness.

Making changes in your life is empowering, but you can expect some resistance from the outside. You may have to upset some apple carts—your own or someone else's. Obstacles to change always arise, but this dynamic tension is actually grist that helps to shape you. That tension marks a creative dialogue between the inner and outer worlds. For true dialogue, you must find your own voice and the fortitude to speak. Let meditation strengthen this ability.

Meditation is like a mini-vacation from your life; you return with a new perspective. Often insights emerge unexpectedly as you go about your activities. Half an hour after meditating you suddenly realize that a relationship is over, or that you've outgrown your job. Someone is taking you for granted, or your needs are not getting met. The time to move or to do the things you've always wanted to do has arrived. This is not a willful choice but an illumination, as when a light is switched on in a dark room.

Sometimes what you realize is that you are not going to change. You have been holding on to dissatisfaction with some aspect of yourself, and all at once you come to terms with it. You are what you are and that's that. You do not really want to be around that person after all, or you just don't like country music. You are not going to lose those ten pounds, and so what? Or you've been thinking that your job is temporary, or that a relationship is disposable. *I don't really live here. Someday I will escape.* But now you see: *I am here. This is who I am. This is my life.* These are simple realizations.

On the other hand, you may have an uncomfortable awakening. Abruptly you see that you have been oblivious to gifts from others and that the time has come for you to give back. Or that you've been resentful, as if dragged unwillingly by life into places where you haven't wanted to go. You suddenly "cop to" that attitude and realize that you have to drop it. Seeing this dynamic in other people is often easier than seeing it in ourselves. When you do admit your resentment, the experience is one of realignment of the self—humbling but deeply powerful.

New behavior arises because you have created the space for change. You have stayed present and listened to all your inner voices, all your guilt and dread. By listening, you have absorbed their power. They have finally gone silent because you have heard everything they have to say, and in that space of stillness you have become a different person. You are changed because you have finally listened to yourself think. This is your inner authority.

Imagine yourself as a queen who sits on her throne and hears the opinions of all her subjects: her consultants, the vizier, the jester, the ladies in waiting, the henchman, the barons and bishops, the midwives and farmers. The old witch from the forest, the elves and fairy people, the beasts and the harpies—all come forth with their pleas. The queen's task is to listen, discern, and claim the sovereignty to speak: "Enough. I have heard you all, and you are dismissed. This is the action that must be taken so that all subjects in my care (self and others) may prosper."

Standing Ground

Sovereignty comes when you inhabit your self, and it has a spatial correlate. You are inside your own skin. Your boundaries are intact. You find your ground and dare to stand tall. You take up space. When you are centered in the self and acting with integrity in the world, we call it "being grounded." You are connected to your inner roots and can stretch out wide and high. You stand in your power and take your place in life.

My feet connect with the Earth.
I inhabit my personal space.
I am a distinct entity in rapport with the life around me.
My individuality emerges in the context of the larger environment.
I know where my place is in the world.
I can deal with life, with whatever shows up.
I am no pushover; my roots are deep.
I am responsive, not rigid.
I can move in any direction at any time.
I can sense when something is not right for me.
I can say no or yes with clarity and conviction.
I can feel in my body all my experience and what I have learned.
I don't need permission to take up space.
I can breathe fully; I don't have to shrink and apologize for being.
I can heartily expand and meet the world with joy.

SOVEREIGNTY WITHIN MEDITATION

Sovereignty means "not owned by anyone else." In meditation, sovereignty means owning and being loyal to your own experience. You give priority to the needs of your inner life. It means you trust your instincts. You give yourself permission to find what works for you and to discard notions that seem alien to you. Your inner authority determines the technique you need each day. You take a supportive attitude toward yourself and accept whatever comes up. You celebrate what an individual you are. You don't make yourself wrong for being different from someone else, or from some generic mold. You learn from your longings and desires. You check things out from your own frame of reference. You take things from the outside with a grain of salt. You know that power resides within. Initiation comes from your own soul, not from an external authority.

As Buddha said, don't believe a thing because it was said by angels, or gods, or saints. Believe only what you have checked out and what works in your experience.

Follow Your Own Trail

Each moment of meditation is an adventure into the self, an opportunity to get to know the regions within. You are following your own trail, tracking your own scent. What you discover and return with from every meditation is some aspect of your essential nature. You are the terrain, and you are your ultimate guide. That is why no outer authority supersedes your own.

The pathway of meditation is not predetermined, and there is no final destination. That's what makes it so much fun. It is more like a meandering journey, full of surprise and delight. It may exalt you to high mountaintops or realms of celestial bliss. It may plunge you into deep forests, into dark caves, or down to the ocean floor. You'll sing with the angels, howl with the wolves, and whistle with the whales. We figure you are the adventurous type—you wouldn't be reading this book if you weren't. So don your favorite gear, lace up some sturdy shoes, and bring your bathing suit!

At certain crossroads on the trail you are likely to see many billboards: "Sign up here, salvation guaranteed!" "Turn here for the fastest path!" "Danger, turn back, follow our ancient way!" "No, over here, ours is even more ancient!" "This is the one true way—you'll never make it without us!" "Enlightenment in three easy lessons! Buy now, pay later!" These messages can be extremely confusing, especially when you're at a turning point in your life, feeling vulnerable, and wondering whether you're on the right track. You may doubt yourself and feel discouraged or lost. But you have the tools you need, right there in your body. Trust your intuition. Follow your nose, your belly, and your heart.

Finding your own way takes courage. It is amazing that just being yourself can seem so bold. It can feel forbidden, like rebellion or even theft, as if you have to steal back your own power. But beyond the "rebellion" is simplicity. When you claim your inner authority, your feet touch the ground one gentle step at a time.

CAVEAT WOMAN

Beware, woman! There are fantasies surrounding meditation and spirituality that may be toxic to you.

Meditation should be based in a woman's own experience and should enrich her daily life. But most of what we know about meditation comes from strict, male-dominated, hierarchical systems that practice external authority and demand that meditators surrender to a God-man who embodies the Truth. These teachings tend to be anti-instinct, anti-ego, and anti-emotion. They may work for monks but can disenfranchise and subtly harm women. If you live in the world—working, loving, and having a family—you need your instincts, your ego, and your passion. They are keys to your inner knowing—not to mention your health. So don't let those stodgy old ideals sabotage your female power.

Watch out for these pervasive notions that are designed to undermine your inner authority: Purity. Enlightenment. Hierarchy. Obedience. Stillness. Detachment. Disembodiment. Dispassion. Control.

None of these have anything in particular to do with meditation. They are part of orthodox religion and monasticism. We present these notions here so that your psychological immune system can identify them and deal with them. If you let them in, they will breed in you like germs. These are particularly potent ideas because so many powerful, celibate, male meditators have struggled with them and propagated them over thousands of years.

The male hierarchy has always taught that spirituality is not in the body but beyond it. God is elsewhere. The body is a trap. Meditation is a discipline imposed from above. It requires obedience to a lineage or a teacher. Meditation is flat and monotonic; there is one right way. Meditation is stillness, not movement. You say no to and attempt to impose silence on your inner voices. You must detach from and block your desires and passions. Meditation is about purity, about getting off the wheel of karma. It is about death.

Now consider the opposite. Nature is sacred. You can meditate from your feminine nature, in the body. Meditation is not a rigid discipline, but the process of answering an inner call. Meditation is the rich inner experience of alternating serenity and passion. It is a great place to listen to yourself think and to tune in to your inner knowing. Meditation is a dance between the earthy and the divine; it is life on all levels. Think of meditation as the integration of opposites—you embrace all possibilities of stillness and movement, purity and impurity, self-will and surrender. You learn to live fully and to let go.

Purity

It is important to extract the basically sound ideas from the truly dangerous. One of the most deadly and confusing centers on purity—the idea that the purpose of meditation is to purify your mind, emotions, and body in order to be spiritual.

Watch out for the suggestion that who you are in your ordinary being is impure, that to be conscious is to be constantly at war with the self. Beware of the belief that your ego is corrupt, your thoughts are disturbances, your senses are illusory, and your emotions are a big mistake, with the possible exception of exalted, detached, and disembodied love. According to this belief, nature is unclean and truth is elsewhere, so you must renounce and transcend your physical self. The body is a noxious bag of excrement and pus (yes, some texts actually say this quite graphically)—especially female bodies with all their disgusting processes. Hence the ascetic practices, violent purging, strange bowel habits, extreme fasting, and rigid diets.

This is bulimic thinking disguised as spirituality. Many women are easy marks for the self-loathing hidden in such teachings because when they look in the mirror that is meditation, they often despise what they see. They hate their emotions and their thoughts just as much as they hate their bellies, their butts, and their boobs. The inner authority to question this knee-jerk response is not cultivated, so ironically, a practice that should lead to a deeper, healthier sense of self actually creates more alienation and even despair. These long-term effects are insidious; they often don't show up until a woman has been meditating for years.

In reality, purification does take place during meditation, as it does in any rest state—you just don't have to think about it. You don't have to instruct your body to get rid of fatigue. In the same way, your mental processes are addressed as you meditate: you confront habitual reactive patterns; you squirm with self-recognition at the ways in which you've been unkind; you see the folly of assumptions you have made. This all happens naturally in the restful spaciousness of your inner world. You don't have to make yourself be good.

What is needed far more than "purification" is quality nourishment and regeneration—a warm and fertile internal climate. Such a female-friendly meditative atmosphere provides the healthful circumstances for whatever must be integrated, faced, or released. Such nourishing also promotes wholeness, compassion for others, and profound connection to the mystery of life. What better "goal" could there be?

Working Against Nature

The emphasis in monastic techniques on efforts to eradicate passion, emotion, and sexuality reflects not just religious idealism but a definite pragmatism. Since many monks enter the hermitage as young boys, they have almost no experience with women. When you are cloistered away with a bunch of men, you learn every trick in the book to avoid being turned on or having desires that would make you stray from the path. Worse, if a monk allows himself to be seduced by one of the local women, as occasionally happens, irate villagers are likely to retaliate. As we were writing this chapter, we learned that a monk in Cambodia impregnated a woman and her neighbors reacted by burning down the monastery!

To understand male spirituality, it is essential to consider how the male sexual organs work. Men's testicles often produce upward of 100 million sperm a day. Give or take a few million. Every second, thousands are coming to maturity, getting ready to go out and swim to meet an egg. An equal number die. Thus, one could say that men have their periods a thousand times a second. Or you could say that men are always lactating. Testicles fizz with creativity.

Nature wants every man to be ready, on a moment's notice, to inseminate all the women on the continent—or at least provide enough sperm to do so. And nature is not easily denied. If a man thinks admiringly of a woman, his body cranks up the sperm and the juices to carry them into her body. If he thinks she is with another man, even more sperm is produced to outdo the other guy's supply.

So for men to be celibate takes some doing. It turns out that if a man can cut himself off from his instinctual nature, he can find brief periods of freedom from the sizzling creative juices. It is a heroic struggle, with nature as the enemy. Thus, spirituality for males is traditionally construed as an inner war, as *opus contra naturam* (work against nature).

Monks may need meditation to be a cool dry room to help maintain their aloofness from life and keep the boners at bay. If women are to be healthy in meditation, however, they must embrace the warm, moist realms of body, emotion, and soul. If you adopt ideas and ideals that were developed for monastic life, it is somewhat like taking medication for a disease you don't have—like taking antibiotics when you don't have a bacterial infection. Many women feel dried up and depressed after years of diligently practicing Eastern meditation, as though they have been led away from their feminine nature.

People have a sense of how to handle the fundamentalism in their own culture. They can join it or not. But when your Eastern meditation teacher starts spouting fundamentalist ideas worthy of a seventeenth-century New England preacher, the message is sometimes hard to decode. The ascetic approach amounts to plastic surgery on the soul—cut, snip, sever the nerves and connections to the passions of mortal life.

In this book we present meditation as a work with nature, an *opera cum natura*. (The Latin term "opus" refers to slave labor, work you are forced to do; "opera," by contrast, is work you *choose* to do, more artful and refined.) Killing off your passion and sexuality is a big loss; it is great for your meditation to be erotically charged. The liveliness and gusto of your erotic life make for more interesting journeys to the inner world, and more integration of transcendence.

Off the Map

Opening to the currents of the inner dance is an experience of direct knowledge, personal and tangible. As you develop your ability to sense subtle energy, stay close to your immediate perception.

Older cultures have formulated maps of energy: the Hindu energy centers in the body, or *chakras;* the meridians or pathways of *chi* in

Chinese medicine and acupuncture techniques; the Taoist principles of balance and flow. Some contemporary teachers have integrated these systems into a broader understanding. For example, Carolyn Myss has correlated the seven Christian sacraments, the seven Hindu chakras, and the *sefirot* from the Jewish cabbalah. These maps engage the mind in valuable ways. But just as most medical experiments and their findings are modeled on male subjects, so too are most of these spiritual blueprints based on an old, male, linear framework. As much as all those concepts may open your mind, they can also predetermine and limit your experience. Notice the ways in which you may be different from what you've been taught. Do not get trapped in the map.

For example, the concept of *kundalini* from yoga and other spiritual disciplines is that the life force ordinarily coiled at the base of the spine is awakened through various practices and eventually makes its way up through the chakras until it bursts in enlightenment through the crown of the head. But energy unfolds in very idiosyncratic patterns, not necessarily sequentially upward. Different centers open as needed according to each person's nature, the essential "stuff" she is made of, her inquiry and passions in this life. There is no one, predictable formula.

Lorin speaks of the current of life energy as a magnetism; it is relational and opens naturally on a need-to-know basis as a person explores being alive. In a group of meditators doing the same exercise, each person's experience is different in response to the challenges of her own life and loves. This is as it should be. The state of enlightenment may itself be very particular to the individual. The intelligence within you is eager to present the subtleties of spirit. If you follow only the map to a predicted destination, you miss the surprising revelations that can only come through open exploration. More important, by trying to engineer the process according to abstract ideas, you may override the innate wisdom of your own system and inadvertently do yourself harm.

The old schema is based on an up-down hierarchy: spirit up, matter down; father up, mother down; enlightenment and freedom up, bondage and illusion down. The assumption that being spiritual means going upward is a tough one to dispel, and it pervades much of our thinking. This schema is archaic and limited, however, stemming from early primitive beliefs that the earth is flat and the sun is a god in the sky. Our relationship to the earth, gravity, and the sun *is* mysterious. But humans can now perceive the cosmos from outside of the solar system, and our internal maps must evolve as well, not by tossing out the old but by becoming more inclusive. Gravity, for instance, is now understood as a relationship not just between our bodies and the earth but between the earth and the sun and moon, between the sun and other stars in the galaxy, and between the galaxy and other galaxies throughout the universe. Gravity is not just a local phenomenon but an omnidirectional, constantly moving field of connection.

Each level of understanding has its place, like Newtonian physics, which still has practical application. But the up-down model of consciousness is static, unchanging, and mechanistic, with no sense of organic movement or surprise. This is why exploration in intrinsic movement, such as the elegant organismic movement of Continuum, is at the cutting edge of perception. There a revolution is under way.

It was a shock when I first physically experienced the field of possibility beyond the maps of higher and lower polarity, beyond local gravity, beyond above and below, at a Continuum workshop with Emilie Conrad in 1983. In the fluidity of subtle movement, the old templates dissolved and a naked freedom emerged: a weightlessness, as if gravity held me lovingly from all directions at once. I was suspended and supported in the embrace of space, in an erotic 360-degree engagement with the cosmos. In this open state was a *knowing* that consciousness pervades everything and is constantly evolving, and that there is no final perfection. I immediately perceived—not as an abstract theory but as a direct impression—that energy and matter are one substance. In this state of unity the whole concept of "spiritual" no longer made any sense; it simply fell away because *it had no opposite.*

That opening undoubtedly came in response to my passionate inquiry into embodiment and spirit. Here's the irony: all the old techniques originally came from someone's spontaneous experience; only later were they codified. The flowing energy of *tai chi,* for example, happens naturally with meditative body awareness. As you stay close to your own inquiry, whatever it is, you will surely be led by your passion to the direct experience you crave.

On early navigational charts, at the edge between known territory and the unexplored, the words "There be dragons" would warn the adventurer of unknown perils. Dragons, of course, personified the Western image of all that was scary and evil and were usually equated with the feminine—nature, body, desire, emotions! Dare to venture over the border. Enter the unknown. Be the territory—not the old map.

❧ TAMARA'S GARDEN

Tamara is thirty-seven, a single woman living in the rural Southwest. "I am a willful and somewhat militant woman, a woman warrior. It is hard for me to nurture myself. So it is crucial for meditation to be a place where I can learn to nurture myself. I have studied with quite a few different monks, and I love and respect them, but they do not know about what a woman needs. I love them because I am somewhat like them—arid and disciplined.

"So many of the meditation forms are about controlling parts of the self, or trying to remake yourself into this very specific image. I go into meditation to know myself, and that means all parts—the bad experiences I have had and all the cherished parts. Whenever I accept any ideal of meditation that is presented by a school I am studying with, it pushes me to cut myself off from the parts that do not fit that image. Why would I cut off any part of myself? When I go to meditate, it is not about shutting the door on myself."

Tamara continues: "For me, this is what I have learned meditation is, after years of study: stand in the center of life and say, 'This is life, this is where I am.' I like to make boundaries around myself—draw circles, or make them with stones in my garden, or set up a tent—I have a spherical tent. I dwell within my boundaries and feel safe. There are times when I need this sense of safety and containment more than anything. When I get that, then I can feel my body more deeply, and I can feel my pelvis.

"Then I watch and feel and hear an interference pattern as all the parts of myself vibrate. It's like watching ripples on the surface of water—the interaction of the aspects of my life with each other. I watch and feel the delicate interrelating of the waves, propagating outward and inward, dancing off the other waves.

"My favorite meditation is to go stand in my garden, with my feet ankle to ankle, and let my hands go in and out from my belly. When I breathe in, they move in toward my belly; when I breathe out, they move outward. Then I just make up my own movements—they come to me spontaneously. I put my attention in my palms, and my mind just dissolves, becomes part of my flesh, and becomes this soft, moist substance. Everything becomes one. When I am in that state, thoughts are like clouds going over the sky. I'm not identified so closely with my thinking anymore."

Spiritual Teachers—What's Really Going On?

You may have noticed that in general men inhabit a kind of entitlement that is foreign to women, a subtle, unquestioned right to exist, a sense of place in the universe. Deep down, women strive extra hard to earn a sense of endorsement and entitlement. Ultimately it's an existential quest, and no one can journey for us. It boils down to this: entitlement comes from within, when we live from our own core.

Spiritual teachers are granted an otherworldly entitlement by the good old boys "upstairs." Even female gurus receive an esoteric endorsement under the auspices of a patriarchal lineage. This gets really tricky for their women students.

You do not need a middle man or woman to contact the deeper realities or to intercede with God on your behalf. If you choose to have a teacher or guru, remember this. A teacher provides a valuable focus and a magnetic center around which people collect, thus creating a collective or community. We crave community, an experience all too rare in our scattered social climate. A spiritual community can give us a sense of belonging and being taken care of. It can relieve the anxiety of finding our own way and the fear of "not doing it right" by sheltering us in the authority of another and in collective spiritual values. The support can be comforting.

As a psychotherapist friend notes, women are in an interesting bind these days. We want the empowerment of handling things on our own, but we also need to feel free to ask for help. There is too much pressure to be doing everything ourselves, too much responsibility thrust upon us. The burden can be overwhelming and exhausting. A teacher relieves the loneliness of carrying this burden by giving you the sense that someone is "there." When a teacher is from an ancient lineage, he seems "loving, very old, and wiser than me," as this same friend confides. A teacher can tell you where you are on the map of known experiences and what to do now. The teacher seems to hold the inner door open because he's already been through it; he is on the other side.

Teachers can transmit energy and wisdom, body to body. But stay alert and do not forfeit your individuality in spiritual conformity. Don't abandon your inner knowing in seeking entitlement from an external source.

Be very careful of dogma. There is a prevailing sentiment that all knowledge has already been discovered, that the best maps have already been made, and that any individual variation is pathology. Most traditions are built around the scary injunction that unless you have a teacher and follow that lineage, you will be in deadly peril. It is remarkable how often this warning is voiced, propagating every time the fear that you could become psychotic or lose yourself forever in delusion. Such may indeed be true in the rigid paths where the techniques are preordained, manipulative, and conceptual—removed from the deep intelligence of the body. But what the monks do not know or believe is that when you stay body-related and learn to follow internal clues, the process is organic and never more than your psyche can handle. By never cultivating these basic skills, the monks can never trust them. Rather than drawing from that resource, they condemn the natural (and more feminine) approach as unevolved, misguided, and vain. Do not buy into this misunderstanding.

Every spiritual collective has a blind spot, a shadow, a dark side that nobody dares to address. Such a collective can be just as dysfunctional as any family. There are many types of teachers, and all have their wounds. They often don't know who their audience is and how the needs and strengths of its members may differ from their own. Many teachers assume that what they have learned is true for everyone. Some embody what they teach; others are living the opposite of what they teach.

Meditation teachers are always in danger of losing track of themselves because the temptation to appear enlightened, to play that role, is so strong. There is an addiction to the image of spiritual perfection. All teachers—women and men both—are continually losing themselves in enlightenment, being hit in the face with their own humanity, and then recovering themselves. The cycle runs in seconds, days, or years. Perfectionist ideals lead to disintegration; they create an inner civil war, a war between the parts of the self. Melt those ideals, and let yourself feel the longing underneath.

Charisma is co-created. It is a relationship, the interplay between the teacher and the attentive and devoted audience. Teachers aren't powerful; they only appear to be. The audience is powerful. Listening is powerful. The attentiveness of women is powerful. Women give a power to the teacher because women are powerful with invisible giving. Devotion is a quiet power, a profound generosity. Because it is the teacher who is shining, everybody forgets that it's the women who are powerful.

There is almost always a hidden hanky-panky going on in a spiritual community that no one is supposed to know about but everybody senses. Some juicy scandal is being justified with a "spiritual" excuse: the guru is giving a female member of the community a special "transmission" (uh-huh), or she's his inspiration for some highly esoteric channeling. What must it be like for these swamis, lamas, and roshis, who for most of their lives have been sheltered in male communities, to be thrust into engagement with our liberal Western culture and surrounded by spiritually hungry, sexually emancipated women? What an electrified atmosphere! Can you imagine the culture shock, the temptation, the challenge?

One woman whose openness and fervent devotion have involved her in many kinds of spiritual teachings was recently at a Tibetan Buddhist retreat with a well-known and well-loved lama. She confessed: "Why don't the people in these communities have stable relationships? They are always looking outside themselves for fulfillment. Why haven't they forgiven their ex-husbands and wives? What kind of practice is that? The lama is married, but says that passion in a marriage cannot last. He has taken up with a young American woman, but nobody talks about the scandal that's on everyone's mind. It's very crazy-making."

In an environment of so much meditation and relaxation, energy in the body naturally wants to flow. It is erotic, and people get turned on. The sublimated sexual charge can be intense in such communities. They do provide a great marketplace, however, for meeting and mating with like-minded people, although women outnumber men two to one. Just beware of the bizarre dynamics.

Bottom line: take what's good and leave the rest. As Krishnamurti advised: Be your own teacher. Be your own disciple.

WHAT IS THE EGO?

Ego comes from the Latin word meaning "I am," or "self." It refers to awareness of your personal identity. Ego is the "sense of the self, especially as distinct from the rest of the world and other selves" (*American Heritage Dictionary*). Ego is the aspect of your psyche that is in touch with both your internal and external realities and can direct your thought and behavior to fulfill your needs.

Ego also refers to a sense of appropriate pride in yourself, or self-esteem. Ego is the relationship between you and the world: you know your position, what your capabilities are, what your contribution is, and what you're worth. The ego is not actually a thing at all—it is the name for the process of relating your inner gifts to the outer arenas where you exercise those gifts.

As with all relationships, there can be imbalances. Many women are excessively humble and consistently undervalue themselves. Sometimes this is called low self-worth. "Egotism" is a sense of self-esteem that is way out of proportion in the other direction, an aggrandized sense of your own importance.

One person's egotism, however, is another person's natural and healthy pride, and you can tell the difference only over the long run. If an intelligent young woman wants to leave the small town where she grew up and go to the university in a big city, some of the towns-people and her peers who are staying in the town may say, "Oh, the local college isn't good enough for you, eh? You think you are too good for us, don't you? Well, you'll flunk out and come back here broke, broken, and begging for our acceptance. We look forward to the day!" In labeling her an "egotist," however, they may just be suffering an attack of envy.

The tender irony is that most people who appear to have too much ego are actually quite insecure and have too little ego. They have not yet developed a core sense of self and realistic self-esteem. They want to be out in the world, but because they are shy or feel inadequate, they pump themselves up and put on a protective shell of bravado.

In some circumstances the language of ego denigration has an appropriate place. An essential part of joining some groups is having your ego "reduced," "broken down," or "killed." When you join the military or a convent, the organization doesn't care who you were on the outside—that person is as good as dead. You are now raw material, so get down on your knees and scrub. Obey instantly. Forget all your personal desires. In the military you swear to uphold the laws of your country and to obey unquestioningly your superior officers. In a nunnery you take vows of poverty, chastity, and obedience. A skilled drill instructor or spiritual supervisor takes you through the process of dying to your old self and being reborn with a new status, as a member of the order. If the process goes as planned, you are glad to be changed—you no longer hold to your old image of yourself, and as a part of the group, you are a new being in a new world of possibilities.

Ego-bashing language is also used in twelve-step programs such as Alcoholics Anonymous and Narcotics Anonymous. If you are a slave to alcohol, drugs, an eating disorder, or any of dozens of other addictions, going through this process of ego denigration can be lifesaving. If your sense of self was such that you endangered yourself or others, or spent your family's food and clothing money on drugs, then you did need to die to that self, and the steps of recovery have led to amazing grace. A sponsor in any of the twelve-step programs can lead you through the process of letting go of your old, diseased relationship with the world.

Thus, in boot camp, in monastic institutions, and in drug and alcohol rehabilitation and twelve-step programs there is a sacred purpose to destroying the ego. The amputation is necessary, a rite of passage into a new life. In the competent hands of a drill instructor or AA sponsor, the destruction of the ego can be a healing operation. You separate yourself from your previous life, renounce it, and become dependent on and subservient to a new authority, making yourself totally open to being reprogrammed and bonding with your new group. But unless you are actually in a twelve-step program under the supervision of a wise sponsor, we suggest that you avoid using the term "ego" in a pejorative sense. This label is very misleading and gets in the way of your development of a healthy sense of self. If you mean arrogant, say arrogant. If you mean insecure and you are trying to cover it up, say so.

In twelve-step language, EGO stands for "Easing God Out." It means "the fear that keeps you separate and keeps you from surrendering to a higher power." Because the twelve-step programs are so profound and have been such an effective blessing for millions of people around the world, their use of the term "ego" has caught on in popular culture. Popular culture, however, is basically about marketing. Marketers realize that ego-bashing language is a good sales tool. They have co-opted AA terminology to make a buck. If they can undermine a person's sense of self-worth, they have a foot in the door to sell him their product.

Thus, we have the oft-repeated spectacle of a self-help guru arriving in a new Mercedes to give a talk to hundreds or thousands of people who have come to hear a lecture on meditation. The self-help guru definitely has a good sense of self-worth—she is being paid $30,000 for a few hours' work. When she says, "Your ego is what's standing between you and God!" she's also implying that your ego is getting in the way of signing up for her next extremely expensive workshop. Many writers of self-help books are in the recovery movement, and quite a few of them have become multimillionaires by appropriating the concepts and tools developed in twelve-step programs and teaching them out of context.

There is a dark side to the techniques of ego reduction: they are also used in cults and brainwashing of all kinds—for example, in Communist reeducation camps and in religious cults organized around a charismatic leader. When someone suggests that you have too much ego, watch out. Too often that person wants to either sell you something or disorient and weaken you so that he or she can manipulate you.

In our experience very few women have a problem with an exaggerated sense of self. The opposite is true: because of their communal, egalitarian instinct, women tend to think they have too much ego even when they don't. Thus, they are susceptible to ego-bashing language and react to it by going in the wrong direction. If a woman succeeds in weakening her ego, others will find her more easily dominated and more gullible and compliant, but she won't become more spiritual. On the contrary, she will find it harder to integrate her own spiritual insights.

John Bradshaw writes about twelve-step programs, and he uses the term "ego" in the way we are recommending here. In *Homecoming: Reclaiming and Championing Your Inner Child,* he writes:

> Your ego must be integrated and functional if you are to survive and cope with the exigencies of everyday temporal life. A strong integrated ego gives you a sense of confidence and control. . . . Once integrated, your ego then becomes the source of strength that allows you to explore your wonder child: your essential self. Paradoxical as it may seem, your ego needs to be strong enough to let go of its limited defensiveness and control. You need a strong ego to transcend ego.
>
> Your ego is the agent of consciousness, the vehicle of communication between your inner and outer worlds. Your ego is the attention that holds all the threads of the web that is you. It is the center of your mandala, the conscious mediator between the different parts and levels of your being. A healthy ego has the resilience to manage and flow with them all. Your ego gives you the strength to make decisions from your deepest values and to act on them with integrity.

Work to strengthen your ego and make it more flexible and appropriate. But whatever you do, don't kill it.

INTIMACY AND POWER

When you inhabit your inner authority, you circulate fully with life. Life force streams through you in a seamless circuit—all the way in, all the way through, all the way out. You receive fully and you release fully, over and over again.

The free flow of energy within the body is an intimate dance with the universe. When you meditate, you experience the power of life flowing through you, the power of your emotions, the power of sexuality and surrender. You are touched in the most private way by the currents of love, stretched on every level by the expansive streaming of life. This can—and should—bring up unresolved issues of intimacy and power. If you ignore them, the habit of holding back remains in place and energy cannot be open and free. This is why meditation must include an awareness of these personal issues, not repress or dissociate from them. Meditating in a healthy way in fact develops your capacity to flow with intimacy and power and to perceive the dance more clearly on every level.

As women we are used to creating and holding space for the people we care about, a generosity that flows from the value we put on relatedness. We tend, however, to shrink our own personal space to accommodate others, or to apologize abjectly when we do not. It may be that women give away their power and then forget that they have done so. Self-forgetting is painful, because the flow of energy gets shut down.

Meditation promotes self-remembering. You can exercise the full circulation of energy and gather back your power. As you pay attention to the fullness of your energy you inhabit space differently and learn to sense the integrity of your own presence. This energy sensing is a direct way to cultivate true power: a body-based knowing that has nothing to do with domination or control.

Male meditation techniques are about control—over nature, over the body, over tenderness and pain. These techniques are yet another way to split off from powerful sensations and emotions—to become less intimate. Because men can be so adept at dissociating from their emotions, a classic struggle between the sexes rages on. How often do we request more intimacy from our husbands? Knowing the value of intimacy, why would we want to meditate in a way that flattens it out? Dissociation is the learned ability not to feel, not to be distracted by longing or pain. Numbing out can have value if you are in a war, in a concentration camp, or being physically tortured. But if your life feels like torture, perhaps something needs to change?

Managing the intensity of life is a challenge, to be sure. You can use meditation to become more conscious or less; the choice is yours. With the joy of consciousness also comes the awareness of pain. You can choose techniques that distance you from pain, or you can choose to enter and transform it. Women intuitively tend to take on more than their share of feelings, proportionate to the degree of dissociation in those around them. Women are like lightning rods that channel emotional energy to the ground. Here's the task. Learn now the high art of *association:* the ability to feel what is yours to feel and to release what is not yours.

All too often in social discourse with men, with male authority figures, or in the dynamics of relationship, a woman quietly recedes. She feels invisible but secretly thinks, *Oh, he's spreading his peacock feathers like males do, let him do it. He needs that acknowledgment, he's actually insecure. Ugh, who wants to fight for attention? It's too exhausting, and I don't really care, it's more important to him.* Or perhaps she just likes the dominance of the male; it makes her feel more feminine and secure. If this scenario sounds familiar, check to see how you handle this issue and track the flow of energy in your body when you do. You may simply be deferring in graciousness and are at peace; surrendering can be restful. But if you tend to forfeit your power and subdue yourself, you may be shriveling up inside or festering. At the other end of the continuum, you may be defiant, toughening your armor and pushing to take your rightful space. Self-assertion is exhilarating, but if you are strident and resentful, you may have forgotten how to receive.

Everyone has personal issues that affect the full circulation of energy. Life is a perpetual opportunity for more connection, clarity, and love, no matter what your level of development. There's no perfect, finished state. Intimacy depends on your willingness to feel and expose your emotional reality, and power belongs to those who can expand and embody what they know to be true for themselves. Both require vulnerability, honesty, and courage. Fear of intimacy and fear of power can constrict you and block your energetic flow. Desperately clinging to intimacy or holding on to power has a similar result. These energy dynamics are revealed not only in relationships but also in the privacy of your inner world. The more you meditate, the more you sense this cosmic tango—and the more you want to let go and join in.

SO WHAT IS FEMALE POWER?

As a species, we probably do not yet know the right use of power. Many men suffer from the tyranny of the old-boy hierarchy just as much as women do. With all the personal, social, and global transformations happening today, models of male power are slowly changing. Concurrently, as the role of women in society advances and globalization expands their possibilities, our understanding of female power is evolving as well.

Power in the world has been based on the ability to manifest. In practice, power has usually amounted to power-brokering—the ability to accept or reject, to control. Men and women who are deemed "powerful" often mete out their approval and wield their scorn so that those around them will "hop to." The threat of rejection keeps people subservient. This dynamic bleeds through into spiritual practices, often as a carryover from early childhood discipline or judgmental religious training—the fear of God, the fear of damnation, the fear of banishment and shame.

If we consider how much the texture of daily life for European and American women has changed just since the 1940s and 1950s we can see how much revision is needed in the language of power. Some religious terminology has been updated to add the merciful feminine ("Mother/Father God"). This helps a little. But most parental models still confine women to the role of child, either the good daughter or the rebellious daughter. Although we all need to stay in touch with our child-self, we must be grounded as adults—and not only through identification with the loving mother archetype.

Claiming power by "developing your inner masculine" is another popular model that, once again, strands women within a male reference and the old rules of the game. This directive is unnecessary and ultimately misleading. Despite the value in some of these models, the problem is that they stop the inquiry at the creaky door of what is known. Why not walk through to the freedom—and responsibility—on the other side?

Fear of the feminine has been a social force from the beginning of the patriarchal era. The raw and chthonic power of female bodies and emotions, especially the bloody and violent process of birth, has for millennia inspired awe and terror in men. Humans seem either to worship what they fear or to try to destroy it. Long ago the mysteries of the feminine were honored. Somewhere along the line in Western culture these mysteries began to be suppressed and ancient beliefs were forced underground. Civilization itself has become almost synonymous with control. The Great Inquisition was the epitome of such dominance and intolerance. Historians estimate that over the hundreds of years of European witch-hunts, between one and nine million "heretics" were killed. Estimates vary wildly and we cannot know for sure. From town records one number is certain: of those officially accused, tortured, and burned for "witchcraft," 80 percent were women.

For more fertile imagery of the feminine, we can look beyond the patriarchal societies in India, Tibet, China, Japan, Greece, and the Middle East today to the earlier cultures that predated them. Ancient Hindu and Tibetan iconography are without a doubt the most highly developed. Intricate and diverse images of female deity are venerated, from Shakti to Kali to Tara—most often voluptuous figures with naked breasts, full hips, and vulvas exposed. Many are fierce and disheveled, wildly brandishing swords with a gleam in their eyes. When such goddesses stretch our concept of female embodiment, we can only say,

Hallelujah! (or rather, *Om Shanti!*). Women are reclaiming the ancient wisdom; let us build on that foundation and keep investigating the true power of women today—now from the inside out.

Inner exploration that liberates female consciousness can slip beyond culturally determined assumptions about the feminine. Meditation is our laboratory, and life is our field for research. With our combined focus on both inner and outer reality, we may be able to peer right through the old veils to discover what lies beyond. What new female archetype are we now ready to perceive?

ᕽ EXPLORATIONS

- In what areas do you feel your authority? Study that feeling.
- In what areas do you like to submit to an external authority?
- In what way do you feel "owned"? Do you like it or not?
- Are you comfortable listening to a friend? Can you be comfortable listening to yourself? Can you spend time alone?
- In what ways do you keep yourself small, hiding what you know?
- In what ways do you puff yourself up, pushing yourself to prove your worth?
- Bowing down is emphasized in Asian traditions. It is part of the culture, something that everyone does all the time. What is your natural movement?

ᕽ SKILL CIRCLE #3:
HOW TO MEDITATE WITH
360-DEGREE AWARENESS

Most of our activities in civilized life direct us to be aware only of the area directly in front of us, but our bodies are designed to be aware in every direction. This section shows how to cultivate 360-degree awareness and peripheral vision for use in meditation and afterward.

You have a sense of easy power when you consciously inhabit space. When you take that awareness into the inner world, a universe of subtle perception opens up.

ᕽ WARM-UP: STANDING TALL

Stand up tall and take up lots of space. Be authoritative; stand your ground. Plant your feet wide and connect with your roots. Feel how the entire body of the earth is beneath you as support. Open your arms to whatever position feels expansive and free. Fill yourself with awareness; spread it all around and through yourself. Let your breath be full and allow your energy to radiate freely outward. How far does your energy extend?

This is a posture of confidence, visibility, and readiness for life. If you come up against your "edge," to a place where you feel exposed, pause and explore those feelings and sensations. Be patient and accept the vulnerability, but encourage yourself over time to stretch out and take up more space.

Six-Dimensional Inhabiting of the Self

First, simply locate yourself in space. Look around and see where your body sits in the room. Become aware of the space above, below, behind, to the left, to the right, and in front of you. Begin to focus on one of these directions and then include the others. Explore with your eyes open and extend your peripheral vision to each side and all around you. Feel the alertness of this broadened perception of space.

Then close your eyes and continue to sense each area. Your eyes may glide as your attention moves. When you do this slowly, you may feel as if you are peering into the inner world of each domain. Which areas are the most inhabited already? Which are the least aware? Awareness is a type of illumination; you may actually see more light or feel a tingling or sense of connection. You can also listen intently in each direction.

Along with an awareness of your physical relationship to space may come symbolic meaning. Here we share some common associations that people have with each dimension, but again, don't get trapped in the map. Notice your own associations and let any imagery come. As with any of the explorations, you may want to make notes in your journal about what you discover. Each realm has a resource for you, and relating to them all gives a powerful sense of wholeness. As you inhabit each space more fully, it is as though you have eyes all over your body.

Above The space above your head extends up farther than you can imagine. This is the realm of the sky, the sun, the moon, and the stars, usually associated with transcendence: the beyond, Spirit, heaven, God, the higher Self; disembodiment; the urge to fly. This direction conveys a sense of the more elevated perspectives on life. Feel the spaciousness and sense of freedom around your head and throat. Physically and energetically, this realm relates to the ability to stand tall, to have vision, to speak your truth. How do you relate to what is above?

Below Drop your awareness down to the area beneath your feet. The space below is often associated with the underworld, soul, depth, roots, foundation, the body of the earth. Some people bring to it a fear of hell or other judgmental attitudes from patriarchal religions. If you find this happening, be gentle with yourself. Explore the feeling and gradually develop a new relationship to the ground and what is beneath. Physically connect to your hips, legs, and feet; feel the weight of your body in gravity. Opening to the space below gives you grounding, humility, and strength.

Behind When you become aware of the space behind you, the energy in your back opens up. You may feel as if you have eyes in the back of your head, or as if wings have spread out from your spine. Associations are varied: the past, ancestors, all that has come before, a sense of support, the mystery of what cannot be seen. This area is also related to our personal shadows—to security or insecurity and the ways in which we hold back from life. In most of us this realm is the least conscious, but when we inhabit the area behind us, with awareness, it becomes a source of power and trust. It imparts a sense of resting back inside ourselves, dwelling within rather than pushing forth. We are simply present and life flows in to meet us.

Left and Right First bring your attention to whichever side has the most energy for you. Look or feel all around that side of space with your inner senses, then shift to the other side. Fill up both sides with your awareness. The left side is often associated with mother, female, intuition, receptive energy, and the right hemisphere of the brain. The right side of the body is associated with father, male, active energy, logical thought, and the left hemisphere of the brain. The range of movement to each side speaks to us about relationship with others, the ability to reach out, to touch and make connection. Heart energy flows through the arms and extends through the hands, allowing us to gather in as well as to give. To increase this awareness, let your arms reach out to each side, then slowly bring your palms together. As left and right sides meet through your hands, there is a sense of inner meeting and wholeness. Through bilateral movement and touch, the two halves of your brain join and communicate as well.

In Front Return your awareness to the area in front of you, where attention usually resides. This realm is associated with the power that calls you forward—goals, the future—and determines how you face the world. Being focused in the front is also related to denial of shadow, not being aware of what secretly trails you behind the scenes. This direction holds the ability or reluctance to release the past, to come out or to retreat and pull back. The front is the obvious, visible world and the realm of consensus reality. Feel your relationship to the space in front. How much energy normally flows forward in your activity?

Now let your attention circulate through all six dimensions. Feel the power and centeredness of that perception. How do you inhabit space? How full and extended can your awareness be?

Connection to the Field

With 360-degree awareness you can also cultivate an aesthetic appreciation of space. "Negative space" is a term from art that refers to the shape of space between and around objects, rather than the isolated shapes of the objects themselves. The balanced relationship between an individual form and its environment is what creates beauty and harmony. Japanese art forms and Zen rock gardens, for instance, reflect an extraordinary understanding of this aesthetic.

When you perceive your own body in relationship to space this way, you feel more in harmony with your surroundings. Your individual shape is always nestled into the shape of space around you. You are never disconnected from the whole. Developing such spatial awareness is an effective way to inhabit your individuality without creating isolation. You can stand your ground distinctly but remain in rapport with the larger context you are in. On a very basic level, you can be yourself and stay connected to all the people in your life.

To get a sense of this right now, pause and look around the room. First take the perspective from inside your head, behind your eyes; look out and see the space around you. Then take a point of view from outside your body and see where you're located in the bigger picture. Just shifting your visual attention this way opens your relationship to space.

Now bring your awareness back inside your body and feel your form, the outline of your skin, and how your shape interfaces with the air, the ground, and the seat.

Next, bend one elbow out slightly, creating an arc between your arm and torso. See the shape of the space between, the curve of empty space from your hand to your underarm. That is negative space. Move your arm slowly and see how the shape changes. Then close your eyes and use your inner senses to tune into the relationship between your body and open space.

Now rest with your eyes closed and continue to sense your body in space. Finally, open your eyes and notice how you now perceive your relationship with the environment.

Expanded spatial perception could also be called awareness of the "field," or ambient atmosphere. In field awareness, space itself becomes alive and imbued with potency—a "field of possibility." Everything is vibration and relationship; nothing is solid and separate. In meditative states the inner senses actually perceive this reality.

Scientifically, we know that the universe we inhabit is "potent space" that is invisibly populated with infinite vibrating waves and particles out of which all form is created. Life is a constant energetic exchange. Each individual body is like a standing wave-form—a nexus of interpenetrating vibratory fields that only appears to be separate and still. From all this movement of energy, every living body generates an electromagnetic field that keeps it in relationship with all other bodies, especially the body of the earth. The biomorphic field of the planet contains, supports, and informs every one of its creatures. In addition, many biologists speak of the morphogenetic field produced by each species—a physical resonance that relays information through the bodies of every member of that group.

We are inextricably connected to our species, constantly influencing and being influenced by other human beings and our environment. This inescapable truth has its dark side. Cognizance of the herd can be a source of comfort, communion, and exhilaration, or it can drive you to distraction, loathing, and fear. You experience this energetic sensitivity all the time, albeit subliminally. When you walk into a room filled with people, you immediately sense the field created by that group, its particular texture and rhythms, and you're comfortable or uncomfortable, happy, excited, peaceful, cautious, or disturbed. You may feel that you can be at ease and have fun, or you may want to run screaming from the room. Your body relaxes into the flow, or your viscera, muscles, and nerves tense up. Emotionally, if you pick up on subtle, shadowy tones not consciously admitted by the people there, you may wonder whether the feeling is theirs or your own. Trust your perception and stay alert—your instincts and intuition are at work. This is the interplay of your "vibration" and that of everyone else in the room, and the more awareness you bring to bear on it, the less you are at the mercy of the situation and the more you can engage it creatively. Consciousness always bestows choice.

Meditation is an atelier for the art of awareness, an inner studio for honing your skills of attention in the outer world. Develop your internal sensing of 360-degree space and field awareness, and you'll find yourself more alert and prepared to meet any circumstances in your life.

MEDITATIONS

Core Breath

This is a powerful breath for connecting to your inner core.

Sit so that your spine is erect but without forcing or tensing. If you are tired, lie down comfortably with your knees bent and feet on the floor. Either position works, but they feel slightly different, so experiment with both.

Take a few minutes to settle and check in. First, establish yourself in space. Look around and see where your body is located. Then bring your attention inside. Become aware of your breath and its natural rhythm, and enjoy this awareness for another couple of minutes.

Now, inhale fully through your nose and pause. Feel the internal expansion. Where do you feel the stretch? As your lungs fill, your ribs separate and your chest lifts and expands in all directions: forward, to each side, under your arms, and through your back. The skin of your chest, waist, and belly gently stretches. Notice the particular sensations you have when you inhale. Then exhale slowly. Do this a few times.

Inhale again through the nose and pause. Now focus on the exhalation. This time, exhale through your mouth and create a hoarse whispering *aahh* sound at the back of your throat. Let it feel and sound primordial (and a little like Darth Vader). Relax your tongue and let it lollygag softly. Empty the breath completely and pause for a moment. Feel how your ribs soften and drop, your solar plexus engages in toward your spine, and your belly hollows out. Each exhalation connects you to your inner core and spine.

As you continue to breathe, place your hands on your navel and feel how they rise as you inhale and sink in as you exhale. With each inhalation, notice how the breath fills all the way through your torso. Each breath lengthens, broadens, and deepens your inner space. Your diaphragm is like a drum skin between your chest and belly, and with each inhalation it bulges down into your pelvis to draw air into your lungs. As you exhale, your diaphragm bulges up into your chest to expel the air. Visualize and feel that movement.

As you continue inhaling and exhaling, explore how the breath opens the central channel from deep inside your pelvis, inside your lower ribs and solar plexus, through the center of your chest, the base and tunnel of your throat, and inside your head, sinuses, and mouth. This breath creates movement through your whole core, so if you get the urge to shift or sway slowly, by all means go with this feedback. Encourage your head and spine to move.

Each time you exhale through your mouth, loosen your tongue a little more. This opens the energy in your throat and simultaneously releases any "good girl" residue. I like to imagine that the root of my tongue starts way down in the muscles at the floor of my pelvis, so that my entire inner core feels fleshy, strong, and connected. This is a matter of taste, so to speak, so find your version of tongue release and power.

With each exhalation, imagine that you expel any toxicity that has lodged in your body. Clear out anyone else's inappropriate thoughts or energies and reclaim the integrity of your being.

Do the breath pattern a few times, then relax and rest with the aftereffects. Then begin again, alternating several times between the core breath and quiet attention.

Meditation on Sovereignty

Step 1 For the twenty minutes of this meditation, claim the sovereignty of your personal space. Create an imaginary sphere around yourself as a sacred and inviolable boundary. How far away or close do you want that boundary? Twenty feet out? Ten feet? Wrapped up right against your body? Is it huge vaulted space, or cozy, close, and safe? Is the outer membrane opaque or translucent? Like fire or steel or glass or skin? Within this spherical boundary, let your energy spread to fill the space, 360 degrees. Invoke a sense of strength, centeredness, and protection, and if an image comes, let it inform you. Meditate with these impressions for about ten minutes. Allow thoughts and feelings to come, but keep coming back to the focus of this sovereign space.

Step 2 Inwardly say to yourself, *My body, my breath, my life.* Repeat the phrase several times, hearing it with your inner ears. Then let the intonation change in some way: pause after each word, slow it down, speed it up. Finally, let the words go and sit in the silent power of sovereignty. Be present to the self.

Gathering Power

Start with "standing tall" (see the "Warm-up"). Shift your attention to the energy in your hands. Let your arms move to gather power from the universe. Bring your hands toward your body and pack the energy into your aura. Then release it back out, sending this gathered energy anywhere you choose. Continue alternating between drawing power in and channeling it out. If you'd like to add breath to your movement, focus on the inhalation as you gather in, and exhale as you release the energy out.

Then slow the movement way down until it eventually comes to apparent stillness. Notice how, as the movement becomes more subtle, the sensations can be even more intense. Pause and breathe with the currents of energy. You can sit or lie down for several minutes to absorb the experience, which may take you into further meditation. When you feel complete, make a gradual transition back to your life, infused with these impressions.

⅋ GOING FURTHER

"I AM" Awareness

This mantra meditation is about the relationship between personal identity and cosmic consciousness—a great mystery. When we inhabit the self fully, we become aware that we exist on many levels simultaneously. The mantra "I AM" celebrates and resonates through them all.

Sit comfortably with your spine lightly upright. Take several minutes to settle in with your eyes open, being aware of yourself in the environment where you are meditating. When ready, invite the eyes to close and for another couple of minutes become aware of your inner environment—how you feel inside.

When you are ready, begin to hear the words *I AM* internally. Say the sound with your inner voice and repeat the declaration again and again. Each time you hear the sound, you affirm your entire being. Let the vibration permeate all through you and bring every part of yourself into its resonance. Affirm your body, emotions, and thoughts, even the places that you don't like or the parts that don't feel worthy. Let the *I AM* sound forth on every level.

Allow the rhythm to change in any way. Sometimes the sound will disappear into a rich and resonant silence. Alternate between sound and silence, as you please.

As the sound vibrates in your inner world, you may have impressions of becoming larger. The perimeter of your personal space may expand. You may feel stronger, freer, more alert. The mantra can be a celebration of your existence. Your awareness may spread out as though you can see in all directions, expanding outward to touch the vastness of the cosmos. You may feel as though your whole body is emanating light in every direction, 360 degrees. The usual bounds of identity may seem to dissolve so that your individual substance merges with the substance of the universe. The sound *I AM* may seem to be uttered by a greater source—the voice of a Divine Presence, the giver of life, your universal self, your spirit, your soul.

Continue with the mantra and periods of silent sensing for ten to fifteen minutes. Then gradually draw your attention back to your "localized" self and the room where you are meditating. Notice how your awareness shifts from the expanded and diffused sense of self and condenses into your individuality again. Spend several minutes letting your attention flow back and forth between the larger space and your personal body, between universality and individuality. Then gently open your eyes and be aware of yourself within the space. Take plenty of time to integrate your perception before you get up to move.

How we define ourselves is a function of how we focus our attention through the many layers of being. Awareness has the capacity to encompass the full spectrum of existence. Inhabit the fullness of self.

The Tree of Life

As human beings, we are aware of our place in the universe and straddle the continuum between animal and divine. Our consciousness is a bridge that translates and exchanges energy between the cosmos and the earth, universally symbolized as the Tree of Life. The spine reflects this connection, channeling life force from the root center at the base of the pelvis all the way up through the crown of the head.

Sit so that your spine is vertical and can move slightly. Bring your awareness to the base of your pelvis, to gravity and your connection to the ground. Imagine your sit-bones and tailbone as roots that reach all the way to the fiery center of the earth, drawing vital energy up into your spine. Stay with this and explore the earth connection as long as you like.

When you are ready, shift your attention to the top of your head and the space above you. Imagine tendrils, branches, or filaments that extend upward into the sky to reach for the light. This can have the quality of connection to the universe or spirit. Another classic image is of a lotus at the crown of the head whose thousand petals open as awareness blooms. For some people the movement is reversed, as though their roots come from above into the top of the head. However you feel this connection, let energy flood into you and feed your entire being.

Now let your attention flow back and forth between above and below. Above and below are both sources of life and nourishment. Feel the powerful magnetism as you are pulled in the two directions simultaneously. As this opens energy in your spine, you may become aware of little places that hold back. Invite them to melt and flow, like the life juice of a plant. As they do, you may feel tiny fluid movements, subtle blossoms of energy. When you spread your consciousness between the ground and the sky, it is as though you merge with the Tree of Life. You take your place in creation. Contemplate this mystery.

After meditating with this for fifteen minutes or so, bring your attention back into the room gradually. Be sure to give yourself plenty of time to reorient. Open your eyes slowly, take some deeper breaths, and stretch your physical body. Then prepare to meet the world with this awareness of life inside you.

The Many-Armed Goddess

Many of the Hindu deities have six or eight arms. Most women are used to multitasking—perhaps you can relate to these many-armed goddesses!

This exploration can be done in almost any position—sitting, standing, or moving on the floor. Just make sure you have room for your arms to dance freely. You may want to put on music that creates a quietly supportive atmosphere for this meditation.

Step 1 Begin by establishing your 360-degree awareness. Meditate with the sense that the cosmos welcomes you as you are now and encourages all that you might become. Invoke the feeling that space itself supports you lovingly from all directions and offers you the freedom to move effortlessly wherever you choose. Take several minutes to open to that invitation.

Step 2 Let your hands rise up and float in the support of space. Now imagine that you have at least one other pair of arms. Starting slowly, begin to touch every inch of air around you with your physical and imaginary arms to inhabit the space consciously. Revolve in all directions, letting yourself unfold gently. With your many arms, dance with the cosmos. Reach out with your whole self to the universe. If you get the urge to move the rest of your body, go with it in any way. Explore this for at least five minutes.

Step 3 Finally, bring your physical arms to rest and visualize that your imaginary arms are still revolving all around you: above, below, behind, to the side, in front. Stay with this subtle sense of engaging with space for several more minutes. Then, as you bring the meditation to a close, slowly open your eyes and take some time to dwell within this perception. Celebrate the fullness and freedom of your energy.

❧ REFLECTIONS

- How do you experience sovereignty?
- What feelings arise as you stand tall and gather power?
- Do you notice any injunctions against inhabiting your full power?
- From what you've read and explored, what helps the most to claim your inner authority and set yourself free? How can you best remind yourself of that when you meditate?
- In what area of your life would you like to inhabit yourself more fully? What message can you remember throughout your day?

❧ SECRET #4
BE TENDER WITH YOURSELF

Finally, home sweet home.
What a relief. This was a day from hell!
Everybody at work so uptight.
That creep on the freeway riding my bumper and honking—
What's with him? World gone crazy . . .
Oh, great, junk mail and bills. Later for that.
I need a shower! I need to meditate!

Whew, that's better, washed off all those bad vibes.
Love this sofa, the view from this window.
Relaxing now, settling down. Deep breath . . .

Good, good, good! Always trying to be so darn good.
Who am I trying to please, anyhow? Mommy? Daddy?
    The Big Judge in the Sky?
Somebody always looking over my shoulder. Go away!
    I don't want to be that "good."
'Course, I'll probably never be good enough. That's what I'm really afraid of.
If they only knew my secret thoughts . . .
Damn, where did I put that chocolate?

Whoa, girl, easy now. Hey, this is my life! And this is my meditation.
    I hereby assert my power.
Okay, so what does that mean? I will live fully and enjoy.
I will endorse what I love. I will learn what works for me.
I will break the rules and set myself free.

So, uh, back to this chocolate.
    What if I take a piece and really, really savor it . . .

Make that my meditation? Yep, I could get behind that one.

Jeez, hope the Meditation Police don't arrest me. Just one little bite?

Oh, good lord, that inimitable smell, so intoxicating it makes me swoon.

Ah, the taste, the nuances of flavor—pure heaven.

I could stay with this forever!

I think I'll just . . . linger, let it melt slowly, slowly on my tongue . . .

Deep breath . . . Mmm, so gratifying . . .

Hmm, that's funny. I don't seem to want another bite. That's a first.

What happened? I had the craving, gave into it completely—with
   awareness—

Enjoyed it thoroughly, and it got . . . fulfilled.

   And I didn't deny myself or feel guilty . . .

There's some kind of secret in that. I'm telling you, sweetie, that's power!

❧ ❧ ❧

BEFRIEND YOURSELF

Meditation is an intimate relationship with yourself, and great tenderness is the key to success. The skills of meditation are essentially the same as those in any healthy relationship: giving attention, understanding, and love. You create a space for honest communication. It is not about domination and control.

Meditation can be like the best friendship you have ever had. If you were talking with a really good friend who loves you, you would naturally open up about whatever is on your mind, anything that is bothering you. You might cry, get angry, grieve; you might confess some secret thought or feeling. You would unburden your heart. Your friend would listen, and you would end up relieved, cleansed, reorganized, healed—maybe you'd even laugh a little. Meditation can be this way too, and you get to be your own attentive friend. You are paying attention to the little piece of the universe that is you.

If you are like most women, you are completely overloaded by life. You work hard: you juggle work and taking care of your loved ones, personal relationships, social obligations, your home, body, phone calls, and chores. Women are masterful jugglers, expert at multitasking. Most of us don't rest enough. Meditation may be one of your main times for self-care, your only private time with yourself.

Discover the gentle art of being compassionate toward yourself in meditation. The word *compassion* is *com* ("with") plus *passion*—to be with your passion and suffering. When you meditate, you are there with all your secrets, your innermost sentiments, your private sensations and dreams. Everything in the background of awareness comes forward, intensely. The busier you have been, the more you will hear thoughts swirling in your brain. You will feel all your needs strongly, your unfulfilled yearnings and desires, all the places where you feel unfinished and rough. When you are intimate with someone, a great part of the joy is being able to satisfy his or her needs. The bonding takes place in this flow and exchange. This is the kind of relationship you can cultivate with yourself in meditation: you meet your own needs and accept whatever comes up. You realize that you are there to learn to tolerate greater intimacy with yourself, to love yourself with all your foibles, wrinkles, and sins.

During meditation your nervous system is engaged in sorting through experiences, transforming the negative into the positive. That is why having thoughts in meditation is healthy. Experience metabolizes whenever your body is resting deeply. Life wants you to thrive and puts your instincts to work for healing. During meditation you invite the process to happen naturally, without conscious interference. If you are very tired, fall asleep if you have time. If you are crying, allow the tears to flow. If you are worrying, give yourself room to be with your worries. Learning to flow with this healing process is a major part of learning to meditate.

There are many experiences that happen during meditation that will make you think you have failed:

- You have a million thoughts.
- Your mind wanders, again and again.
- You come back to yourself with a jolt, realizing that you forgot you were meditating.
- You replay conversations that did not feel quite right.
- You feel totally lazy.
- Your posture slumps.
- You fall asleep, for a few seconds or minutes.

- All your bad feelings about yourself come to the surface.
- You feel the tug of longing and desire.

Many people think that these are sure signs of failure, that meditating is a matter of concentrating to make your mind blank. The opposite is true. You haven't failed when all this happens. Your brain is doing necessary housecleaning, making your needs known so that you can tend to them. All these experiences are symptoms of success in meditation—it means you feel safe enough to let go and be yourself.

The simple key is this: accept all your thoughts and feelings as part of meditation, without any reservation. Don't even protest a little. Incorporate this one insight, and your meditation will be much easier. For one thing, your brain will have less work to do because when you have a thought, you won't need to have the second thought: *That thought should not be there.*

Thought has weight and texture. Become interested in the texture of your thoughts, how you touch yourself internally. Many women have more compassion for others than they do for themselves. When they meditate and begin to become aware of their thoughts, they realize how harsh they are with themselves. They tend to take a heavy hand, poking and prodding themselves inside: *What's the matter with you? Can't you pull it together? You're always falling short! Do more. Try harder!* There's always something wrong, some ideal to live up to, yet another reason to manipulate and control the self. Remember Annette Bening's character in *American Beauty?* "Just shut up, shut up!" she exhorts herself, slapping herself in the face, hating her vulnerability. Her pithy display of the internal reality of many women also shows the shadow side of self-improvement schemes—they can provide more fuel for self-blame.

Instead of maintaining such a prickly, pressured texture, consider touching yourself with attention that is delicate, accepting, and kind. Imagine how soothed you would feel inside. Imagine the relief and relaxation. Imagine the sense of inner space, the freedom of your breath, the softness in your heart. The word *attention* has the same root as the words *tenderness* and *tending.* Meditation is the art of attention; you tend to your internal world, as you would a garden or young child. So when you meditate, pay attention to yourself with tenderness. Developing a soft inner touch—and tolerating so much tenderness—

may take a while. But as you become familiar with the sensations, this quality of awareness will soon be second nature. Over time you will find it easier to be tender during meditation and to maintain that approach more consistently throughout your day.

If you are usually very disciplined and goal-oriented, you may find it challenging to soften and let go in meditation. Being tender may seem too warm and fuzzy, too sloppy, or even heretical. You may even fear that a lightning bolt will zap you from the sky. The more advanced you are as a meditator, the more difficult this may be, particularly if you are trained in Zen, yoga, or other very stylized forms. And if you love physical disciplines, if you are a professional dancer or yogini, for example (I am both, so I know whereof I speak), you may be used to working on your alignment every minute of the day. To allow yourself not to work in meditation, to be physically released instead of perfectly in place, may seem virtually impossible. Experiment with the meditations in this chapter and cultivate "Soft Posture" awareness, as described in the skill circle. Notice what thoughts come up as you invite yourself to be physically and mentally tender. You can return to your work stance later, but during meditation, let go. Use your discipline to focus on soft inner touch. Try this for, say, three twenty-minute sessions and see what happens. Go on, I dare you. You will be astonished at the quality of relief, and as energy flows more freely, your alignment may even open in unexpected ways.

When you meet yourself with softness, your internal climate changes. The bitter or acidic inner pH is neutralized. This is a metaphor for very real material changes. Tenderness, compassion, and pleasure are not just abstract ideas; they are sources of physical nourishment and healing. Research validates the impact of the texture of thought on the body. In states of flow, brain chemistry shifts and restorative hormones are released and flood through your whole system. Within seconds your immune response is heightened. If you simply remember a time when you've been loved, or touched by someone's kindness, you can probably recall this subtle internal effect and re-create it just by having that thought.

Cells are in a constant process of regeneration as some die off and new ones are formed. It is said that your entire body is re-created every seven years. Tenderness engenders a transformative and fertile climate for the growth of healthy new cells, for the rebirth of your body from the actual substance of love.

A Moment to Love

Let's pause right now to explore this. Bring to your awareness someone or something that has moved your heart—in love, joy, sorrow, or inspiration. What was it that touched you so? How does that experience still move in you? Your response reflects your ability to see and appreciate—your willingness to be open to life. As you recall the experience, let the feeling flood into the present moment. Notice any subtle physical sensations of release and warmth and recognize them as the nourishing and healing substance of love. Consciously breathe in that loving atmosphere.

INNER TYRANNY

Just as outer relationships can be abusive or disrespectful, the inner relationship can be brutal. Some of your internal dialogue may be blaming, shaming, and fault-finding. As your body settles down, sooner or later you'll notice any self-critical thoughts that orbit around on your periphery. You will also become aware of the effort of holding them at bay. Negative thoughts don't just pop up during meditation. They are already there in the background, and as you become quiet you hear or see them.

Again, women seem particularly vulnerable to suggestions that something is wrong with them, and this tyranny shows up in their internal voices. Why? Perhaps because of the three-thousand-year effort to get women to shut up and behave. Or perhaps because women are so used to listening.

Every woman's heart is in an ongoing conversation with life. Because we are so relational, we are open to other people's opinions, including their critical thoughts. This carries over to the inner world: we hear negative internal voices and tend to believe them. If our sense of self is strong, we may be able to avoid buying into the shaming thoughts and to put them in perspective. But even so, when we are stung by a vitriolic comment, penetrated to the quick, it can take some work to detoxify.

The same is true within. Particularly when you're tired or hormonal, your threshold of vulnerability may be lower and your inner voices louder and more convincing. These are times when you need to be vigilant, to simply witness, to not be seduced by the shame.

Abusive relationships are inappropriately controlling relationships. You do not have to control or edit yourself in any way when you meditate—not even your negative thoughts. Remember to let your meditation be a pleasurable sense of bathing in your own essence. The stereotypical rules of meditation are eerily similar to the repressive voices of some of our parents and teachers: "Don't have needs! Pay attention! Don't wiggle! Keep your hands to yourself! Don't fall asleep! Sit up straight! Have good thoughts! How dare you think or feel that!" These are not the rules of meditation; they are the rules of kindergarten, monasteries, and church. When you find yourself feeling guilty, inadequate, ashamed, or like a failure, know that you have simply encountered one of the erroneous rules. Take a breath and keep going. How do you keep going? Practice "not being mean to yourself." Simply return to your focus, which is something pleasurable, an aspect of life itself.

It's tempting to think of meditating as pushing hard to keep thoughts away. Many books and teachers promote this aim. You must try harder not to have thoughts, they say, because to have thoughts during meditation is to fail at it. You have "monkey mind" (an oft-used slam in Buddhism)—thoughts that play and jump around. This sounds logical to our controlling mind; of course you are supposed to stop thinking to meditate. The model underlying this attitude is that of the ego as a heroic figure striving mightily to discipline unruly thoughts, like Hercules reaching out with his strong arms to fend off the enemy. (What's so bad about monkeys anyway? They are great survivors.)

When you meditate, you are doing something that human culture has thousands of years of opinions about. So your inner abuser has centuries of ammo and justification. The way "self-flagellation" can show up varies from moment to moment. You may feel that you have to sit cross-legged even though your knees hurt. Change your posture and sit comfortably. You may feel selfish or ashamed for having desires and needs; perhaps you feel bad about having angry or sexual thoughts during meditation. Just stay there and feel.

Some of the little voices of shame and blame try to cloak themselves as your inner guide: "I am the Voice of Authority, I am the Voice of Buddha, I am the Voice from On High calling you to The One True Path." One of the patriarchal ideas is shame about being human. Shame leads us to try to "overcome" or transcend our humanness by being perfect. Whenever you feel inadequate or ashamed of yourself just for existing, this dynamic is at work and you need to be alert to perfectionist ideals. The meditation literature is absolutely full of perfectionism—sit perfectly straight, don't fall asleep, don't let your mind wander, be devoted to your guru, be a vegetarian, never get angry, always be compassionate.

When you witness these thoughts and don't let them complicate your approach to meditation, then you win. Each time you do not run away from a "bad" inner feeling, you win back your freedom just a little. The way out is simply to keep on paying attention. When you continue to be there, your attention absorbs and then disperses the bad feelings that have been blocking your ability to entertain cheerfully your own desires.

Internal strictness has nothing to do with meditation. If you buy into a stern discipline, making meditation difficult, you will most likely quit. To meditate successfully, you must give up puritanical rules and replace them with the rules of friendship:

- Don't hit yourself.
- Don't make yourself wrong.
- Don't shut yourself up.
- Don't squeeze yourself into an ideal image.
- Don't delete or condemn parts of yourself.
- Do be tender with yourself.

How to Listen

The technique for dealing with shaming thoughts is simple: you listen, you witness, you feel, but you don't let the critical voices fool you. They are just tape loops your brain is playing, and the meditation process itself steals their power and returns it to you for use.

Realizing how violent we are to ourselves can be a shock. When you hear such thoughts, you probably flinch, but understand that your brain is seeking to heal itself from the fragmentation. As you notice how the thoughts seem to attack you, and how tired your mental muscles are from holding them off, then you become aware of what your inner situation has been. Acknowledging this battle can be painful. The technique of meditation is not to push even more or to shift your footing—like Hercules—to keep this awareness out. The technique is to pay attention to the situation and bring compassion to both sides of the dialogue: the you who is thinking negatively of yourself, and the you who is trying to hold those thoughts away so you can function. Your meditative awareness delicately touches both parts and begins to heal the split.

- Listen carefully to yourself.
- Hear the tone of voice of the thoughts.
- Notice the labels you use to judge your behavior.
- Watch your internal images.
- Feel the sensations.

Now for the antidote: without denying the negative voices in any way or trying to get them to shut up, return to pleasure, return to home base, return to life. Imagine yourself bathing in something positive, something essential to life: breath, sound, light, love.

Listening to the negative voices relieves the inner tension they have created in you and breaks their hypnotic spell. In the fairy tale of Rumpelstiltskin, the beautiful maiden must guess the name of her captor in order to free herself from him. Similarly, listening to and naming your negative inner voices transmutes their subconscious power.

We have compiled some of the mean internal scripts to which women are subject. Sometimes the thoughts are obvious, and sometimes they are subliminal, just below the threshold of awareness. Either way, they are toxic and create an internal climate that is bitter, sharp, cold, and dry. By naming them, we begin to dispel their hold:

- *I really blew it with so-and-so.*
- *I'm always blowing it.*
- *They hate me.*
- *I'm inadequate.*
- *I'm weak.*
- *I don't really know what I'm doing.*
- *I never think of the right thing to say.*
- *I always say the wrong thing.*
- *I'm not smart enough, and nobody likes me.*
- *I'm too smart, and nobody likes me.*
- *I'm too much.*
- *I'm not enough.*

- *I'm ugly.*
- *I hate my body.*
- *I'm too fat (too thin, too tall, too short, too old, too young).*
- *My nose is big (my eyes are puffy, my skin is bad, my hair looks dumb).*
- *I'm disgusting.*
- *I am not fit for public consumption.*

Then it all gets compounded with:

- *I shouldn't be thinking this.*
- *I shouldn't be feeling this.*
- *Stop it, stop it, stop it!*

Because of our relational nature, the most effective attitude to take with these voices is to relate to them. The heroic method of blocking them out or suppressing them does not seem to work for women (if it does for anyone). The voices don't just go away; they remain in the shadows of the subconscious and find clever and diabolical ways to wreak havoc there.

You are not evil, weak, or less evolved for having negative thoughts; everybody has some version of them. But relating to your inner voices without repressing them or being possessed by them requires ego strength; this ability, like a psychic muscle, gets stronger and more resilient with use.

You have several choices of strategy. Each meditation secret sheds a different light on ways to bring consciousness to the inner world and establish a healthy inner environment. Here are some to choose from:

- Listen and simply return to your focus of pleasure and tenderness. In this chapter we focus on cultivating a soft, compassionate inner touch and a sense of flow.
- Realize the erroneous rules you are up against (see "Secret #3: Claim Your Inner Authority").
- Identify the desire behind the thought. Often the critical voice wants us to excel and be our best. Underneath its cruel style is the desire for something very basic, like love or power. Behind "I hate myself" might be "I want you to love me." Because such feelings

&⊗ **MARLA'S STORY**

Just to show how insidious internalized shame can be, here is the story of a woman who has been meditating for thirty years. Marla is well rounded and competent, makes many of her own clothes, and owns several homes. Just recently, on a walk with a friend, she admitted that she doesn't like a certain best-selling book about meditation and healing. She bought the book and tried to read it for a year, but always put it down with a bad feeling after reading a page or two.

While talking to her friend, she realized: "The teachings in the book are irrefutable statements of opinion. It's not an invitation to explore, it's an authoritarian rant. I feel wrong, inadequate, and guilty, talked down to, just like being in church." Instead of endorsing her, the book made her secretly think that there was something wrong with her. Even though she is articulate and well versed in spiritual work, Marla realized that the book "made me feel bad, but I thought, 'Oh, it's me. If I weren't deficient, if I were more evolved, this book wouldn't make me feel bad.' So I feel inadequate for feeling inadequate!"

Be very alert to what makes you feel, "I'm not up to it. I'm not good enough." Your nervous system is a kind of operating system, and some programs will make it crash. You can sort this out by learning to follow what feels good. Take your own side. Eventually you will get past caring whether the criticism is true, and simply be yourself.

This story points out how important it is to have friends who share your interest in meditation but keep an open mind and are not true believers. It is especially necessary to speak with other women and find your own language for experience. Together you can discover hidden beasts of shame and defang them.

are so primitive, it is easier to be self-critical than to tolerate the true longing. (Learn how to enter the desire in "Secret #6: Answer the Call.")

- Name the voice as a character in your "Inner Theater." Learn how to relate to it with curiosity, letting the voice tell you about itself; you can even direct it (see "Secret #8: Say Yes to Every Part of Yourself"). This is an extremely informative exercise. It also transforms the voice into vital energy and sometimes even into humor.

- Remember your creaturehood. Address the instinctive need to which the voice is alerting you and fulfill it (see "Secret #2: Honor Your Instincts").

- If the negative thoughts inexorably pull you down and you feel depressed, the time has come to excavate the treasure below. Learn to descend consciously (see "Secret #10: Do Not Fear the Depths").

- If the criticism is directed toward your body, see "Secret #11: Love Your Body" for support in breaking that cultural trance.

- Keep developing your home base in pleasure (see "Secret #1: Celebrate Your Senses").

THE TEXTURE OF LIFE

Tenderness toward yourself is incredibly sweet. Though you crave gentleness—and everyone does—the sweetness of it can be hard to take. It seeps right through your protective crust, all the way down to your core. Your whole being, body included, warms in that sweet nurturance, and the frozen, untouched places deep inside begin to thaw. As you melt, don't be surprised if tears seep out as well. Cherish the tears. They are the water of your soul.

With the soft touch of inner compassion, the texture of outer life softens as well and the world suddenly seems more compassionate. Your belly and chest breathe more freely, and you soften into your core. Because you begin to live from the inside out, you are bathed in your own atmosphere no matter where you go. With every breath you drink in the sweetness and your entire body is saturated with tender joy. Without any effort or adherence to abstract rules, you radiate tender joy for others. Sensing this, people respond in kind, and even chance meetings in the market or street can be rich with heart. You are permeable, connected, and available for life. You have melted into the stream of love that pulses through every body, the unchanging reality behind the changing shapes. Like a river pulled toward the ocean, you glide into deeper waters, the eternal beneath the passage of time. Slowly, quietly, tenderly, you slide home.

THE INNER DANCE

Circulation

Call it life force, *kundalini, chi, ki,* spirit, *shakti,* or *prana,* it is the unimpeded circulation of energy that gives us health and satisfaction. When we soften to ourselves, the internal pathways open and energy streams through us more fully.

Life is generous: it wants to flow through us amply and freely. To surrender to the sensations of this much physical and emotional movement is a big deal. Learning to increase your capacity to sense energy and to tolerate more current surging through you takes time. It is a gently progressive, inclusive process, and that is the practice. Your nervous system gradually gets used to "higher voltage"—more electromagnetic energy dancing through you, as you.

Like sex, exercise, and deep breathing, meditation promotes full circulation and is revitalizing. Here's one advantage of meditation: you get to be outwardly quiet so that you can inwardly track the currents and enjoy them even more. This inner sensing is the basis of many healing practices.

The body in its wisdom naturally opens and balances energy if we do not interfere. The secret is to cooperate with the process and provide the right environment. Staying physically and emotionally fluid is key, and awareness is the magic ingredient. We do not have to engineer or control; in fact, it is mostly about letting go of control. This principle is one of the most important foundations of this approach to meditation. If you can embrace this simple truth, you'll save yourself a lot of angst.

❧ THE RIGHT TO SWOON

A meditator for almost thirty years, Theresa has practiced many different forms. At one point a few years ago she was at a retreat with a famous Indian woman guru. Everyone was meditating to a sensuous chant, and the guru swooned and moaned in ecstasy. Theresa too could feel the rapture and began to sway with the chanting.

When she opened her eyes, people were glaring at her disapprovingly. Later a leader took Theresa aside and said, "We don't do that here. You are distracting people." Apparently, only the teacher was allowed to surrender to passion.

What is so sad about this is that for Theresa this kind of devotional surrender and dancing is the perfect fusion of body and spirit and would have been deeply healing for her. Faced with a heart-rending choice, Theresa decided to leave the group. This is an example of how meditation groups lose women and the contribution of their natural wisdom. Women always come up with wonderful ideas, but too few of them are accepted.

Spontaneous movement often happens when you sit to meditate. It is to be welcomed and enjoyed. Like Theresa (and the woman guru), claim your right to swoon.

Everything Is Flow

When you meditate, it's often nothing like stillness. The experience is more like a dance, an inner swirl of movement. Life is flow, not stillness. Breath flows, blood flows, emotions flow, thoughts flow, rivers flow, music flows. Even atoms and molecules are always vibrating. People associate meditation with stillness, but the techniques are actually about entering the flow more deeply: the flow of a mantra, the flow of breath, the flow of thought, the flow of currents of energy. That there is stillness somewhere, and that we should stop moving, is an illusion. During meditation we sometimes have sensations of total stillness, and it is so sweet an experience that we mistake it for fixity. But the sensation is like a car moving on a smooth highway, or the propeller on a fan being perfectly balanced: the quality we crave in stillness is balanced flow, harmony, and grace in motion.

The stunning truth is this: we *are* flow. "We do not do movement, we are movement." The revelation behind this succinct statement by Emilie Conrad has revolutionized the field of somatic studies and healing. You are flow, at a spiritual, physical, emotional, and subatomic level. This is not just a metaphor but a tangible reality that you can learn to sense. To experience this flow is ecstatic (literally, "out of stasis").

Everyone, of course, holds on sometimes, and every body has its habitual ways of getting tense. When you meditate, you can realize how you have been holding tight, then soften into the rhythm and flow underneath the tension. As you relax, your blood vessels dilate, your circulation is enhanced, your blood pressure decreases, and your nervous system balances itself. There is a palpable release as pathways of subtle energy open up—an actual *gush* of pleasure. You sense the dance that is going on—and has always been going on—as an ineffably sweet pulsation of life, as waves of fluid, as a gentle pumping of lymph and blood through the veins. Join this movement and be led to the stillness at its core.

The Big Secret About Emotion

A woman's emotional body is astonishingly fluid. As you let go into flow, your meditation may at times be a wild internal ride through many different emotional tones. The great art is to participate in all the flux. Integration comes from the full movement and accessibility of all the emotional qualities, not from a bland and static calmness. Equanimity is the equal acceptance of all parts of your soul.

Think of "e-motion" as "energy in motion." When the nervous system, the psyche, the spirit, the body—choose your phrase—has the freedom to unfold, the fertile spectrum of energy that we call emotion reveals itself in all its colors, glory, and gore. When we learn not to suppress the flow, the energy shifts spontaneously and quickly from one tone to the next. Each surge is emotional in flavor but does not need to have specific content, nor does it even require a label—anger, sadness, fear. The whirl of energy may not be about a particular issue, memory, or personal statement but more like the weather—the expression of a life force that simply must have room to move.

Because women's access to this fluctuating elemental energy can both terrify and inspire awe, its secret is a feminine mystery. It is the volatility and unpredictability of primal energy that terrify the uninitiated. Most men do not experience this energy, and many women also fear its power, for understandable reasons: all too often elemental energy has been usurped, misapplied, and acted out in blame or rage. But it can also clarify, liberate, and inspire. That is its purpose.

This is demonstrated clearly when we take meditation into spontaneous movement. When we surrender to the flow of energy and ride the currents consciously, we are plunging into the creative torrent of life. We are carried in the timeless stream and actually shaped by its primordial power. An archetypal force beyond our personality moves our bodies, our voices, our breath. The myriad faces of the Goddess appear through us—sometimes tender, sometimes raw and fierce. For that second, minute, or hour, we become Her—we are all of Her faces, and none of Her faces. We cannot hold on to any of these evanescent revelations, but we can witness and participate. We flow, and we are washed clean.

&ent; EXPLORATIONS

- *Be a friend to yourself.* What qualities of attention would you want from a good friend? Discern how you would like to be listened to, then practice giving that kind of attention. You can practice with your friends—listen with total attention and unconditional love for twenty minutes to someone you care for. You can practice with strangers you fall into conversation with. Attend to yourself in the same way during meditation. Learn about intimacy with yourself.

- *Identify your habitual self-criticisms.* What are your most common negative thoughts about yourself? When do they come up most often? What is your usual mode of dealing with them?
- *Remember times when you have felt soft and tender.* Maybe it was after having a good cry, receiving a massage, or making love. Did the experience change how you perceived yourself or the world?

❧ SKILL CIRCLE #4:
HOW TO MEDITATE WITH FLOW

Energy unfolds through compassion, not discipline. We tend to be cruel to ourselves and to internalize any negative voices we have encountered in our outer world. Meditators have to be alert to this tendency and not let critical voices take over the meditation technique (they will criticize us for not meditating right). A lot of the noise of meditation is feeling through all the ways you've been mean to yourself during the day—bullying or betraying yourself.

Develop a soft touch in meditation. Get used to continuous movement on all levels all the time. Don't try to impose fixity on yourself—add Lycra to everything. Creativity depends on flow; it cannot emerge in an atmosphere of constraint. The parts of you that know how to play can bring more freedom into your meditation. The parts of you that are tender know how to be moved. The willingness to be moved is a secret of the heart and leads to inspiration and joy. Cultivate this willingness. Be moved by love, be moved by your soul, be moved by the spirit of life.

"Soft Posture" Body Awareness

People often take a military stance to meditate—mentally and physically. Even if you are in the military, there are always times when you can be "at ease." Whenever we hold a position, we tend to cut ourselves off from deeper movement. Instead, relax into openness.

Most meditators think they should be stock-still and erect. They have heard that meditation is about opening energy in the spine, so they valiantly try to sit up straight. Their rigidity actually impedes the flow

❧ WARM-UP:
SOFT TOUCH

Experiment with soft attention right now. Pause and take a conscious breath. How tender and loving can it feel? Bring your fingertips to your face and lightly touch your skin and feel how delicate and sweet that touch can be. Can you feel your internal climate beginning to change?

that would allow the energy to open. The other name for *kundalini* is "serpent power," because it moves in subtle, snakelike waves through your core. Undulation may be second nature for people from India (have you seen those wonderful head wiggles some Indians do when they speak?), so perhaps it just never occurred to the yogis to talk about letting the spine move.

Sit softly upright so that your spine can be fluid and free to sway slightly. Your head can just float on top. Place your feet on the ground, or fold your legs up if that's a comfortable position. Some people like to sit on their heels with a *zafu* or pillow propped under their bottom. Find what is most natural for you. Bring awareness to your face; soften your eyes, your lips, your tongue; separate your teeth slightly so your jaw releases. Your hands can simply rest on your lap or thighs, palms relaxed and facing up or down.

When you meditate, you probably notice little places of tightness. Touch them with awareness; imagine that your breath is caressing and soothing them. The flow of breath is like an internal massage that gently opens you up, so give yourself the freedom to go with its wavelike movement. As your body releases tension, it makes tiny shifts: your shoulder drops, your ribs soften, your spine undulates subtly, your head tilts. Just keep allowing yourself to be soft. Invite yourself to melt inside, to spread open in every direction. Rather than a vertical act of will, opening up this way feels more like the concentric ripples of a pebble in a pond, or the delicate unfurling of the petals of a rose. With each opening there is a little gush of pleasure, a "yes" or "mmm" from your body. Slowly and gently, your holding patterns unwind and you ease into fullness.

A supportive context helps to let your body surrender. A group environment provides a larger and stronger energy field, especially when some of the other bodies already know the fluid inner realms. Continuum movement meditation, for example, is a wonderful group context, so if you ever have the chance to take a workshop, plunge in.

Spontaneous Movement

As you get used to "Soft Posture" awareness, you bodily experience yourself as flow. Notice the impulses to move and cherish them. When you don't hold on, spontaneous movement is right there, however subtle. As you yield to the sense of flowing motion, it's as though you are floating in a warm and friendly ocean. In deep meditation your body may lean or sway, your fingers may spread in little gestures, your hands may even rise up and drift through space. Your breath rhythm may change, and your eyes or mouth may take on different subtle expressions. You may find yourself doing an improvised *tai chi,* because this is the original responsive state from which those movements were choreographed. As you give over to the flow, your body does an intuitive balancing of energy, your personal *chi gung.* It can feel mystical but totally natural. When the movement carries you this way, you know there is no separation between you and the divine dance of the cosmos.

Floating Hands

Anytime you get a hankering for spontaneous movement, you can intentionally help it along. Use subtle music as a background ocean of sound; this encourages the feeling of support in space and provides the inspiration to move. In addition, experiment with "Floating Hands." At some point in your meditation, allow your hands to rise up gently into the space before you as if in buoyant water. Just lift them slightly off your lap so that the weight of your arms is suspended. In this way you signal your body that you are ready and willing to swim.

Sacred Gestures

In movement meditation you sometimes find yourself in one of the sacred gestures, or *mudra.* You have seen these mythic hand movements in classical Indian dance and sculptures of the gods and goddesses. When this happens in meditation, it is as if you have spontaneously tapped into the biomorphic field of a timeless archetypal ballet.

The way the hands merge in prayer is a mudra. Reaching out with open palms is a mudra, as is touching your own heart. Explore various expressions of the hands and notice which ones are satisfying to you. For example, draw your thumb and another fingertip together, fan your fingers out, and tilt your wrists or elbows to different angles. Play with separate moves for your right and left hands, as well as symmetrical shapes. If you find a gesture that speaks to you, use it intentionally in your meditation. Breathe with the feeling tone evoked by that sculptural shape, with the energy flows within it, with the expression and poetry of the pose.

You can also start with two or three choreographed gestures and flow from one to the next, letting yourself be surprised at what happens in between.

Stability and Fluidity

Every woman has her own balance between stability and fluidity, structure and freedom, planning and spontaneity. Recognize and accept the mode you prefer. If you follow your innate preference, you may gradually be drawn to its opposite. An analogy is the complementary relationship between yoga and dance. While both create strength, centeredness, and flexibility, yoga focuses on structure, stillness, and inner calm, and dance on spontaneity, mobility, and expression. Eventually you will find your synthesis between the two modes. As our friend Shiva Rea, a well-known yoga teacher in Los Angeles and writer for *Yoga Journal,* has discovered, "If I didn't have the wildness of African dance, I would never be able to do the discipline of yoga."

MEDITATIONS

All of these meditations are enhanced by the addition of subtle and gentle music. Listening to the soft texture of sound is one of the most effective cues to your nervous system to let go.

Breath of Compassion

This exploration of the exquisite tenderness of the breath is marvelously simple, and deeply regenerative. First take a couple of minutes to settle in, letting your eyes close if they want to. Invoke the space to be with no demands on yourself whatsoever. Then become aware of your breath, just as it is. Notice how it flows without any will or effort on your part, in from the air around you and back out. Let the rhythm establish itself—no need to change it in any way. The breath may be shallow or deep, extremely slow or rapid; it may pause as if forever when you exhale.

Now bring your attention to the texture of breath, how soft it is. Feel the tenderness brushing through your nose and throat, the gentle swelling inside you with its accepting touch. How soft can it be? Intentionally surrender to the tenderness; dissolve any judgment and pain. Know the abiding movement of breath as the spirit of acceptance within you. Receive the blessing. Breathe with compassion for yourself.

A Gentle Awakening

This short meditation infuses your first waking moments with self-remembering and sets you up with a beautiful tone for the rest of the day. Do this for five or ten minutes in the morning before you get out of bed. Afterward do the scalp massage and some of the easy stretches before you rise (page 266).

Lie on your back comfortably. Bring your right hand to your upper chest and your left hand to your lower belly. You will feel the exact spots that call out for contact.

The soft touch of the breath inside meets the soft touch of your hands. Breathe into that contact and let the energy soothe and nourish your belly and heart. Pay attention to the subtle feelings of warmth, release, and comfort and let them remind you to be tender with yourself. Drench any anxious thoughts with compassion and imagine moving through the day with this quality of acceptance and care. As you focus on the sensations of caring attention, you gently awaken into the atmosphere of love.

Heart in Hand

Sitting comfortably, take plenty of time to settle in. Then gently rest your hand on your heart. Breathe into the place of contact between your hand and your chest. Feel the warmth and energy, as though a subtle message flows back and forth between your palm and your heart.

Slowly move your hand away, and then even more slowly return, as though magnetism draws your hand back to your chest. Receive the touch again. Feel the communication of energy again. What is being said?

Repeat this motion several times, moving away slowly and returning. Allow the sensations and emotions of coming home to your heart.

❧

❧ GOING FURTHER

Sway Away

This is a very relaxing exercise that can be done with soft music if you like. Sit comfortably and take a few minutes to become aware of your legs and pelvis. Appreciate how your upper body flows softly upward from that base. Begin to sway through your torso, gently shifting your weight side to side. Your spine will become liquid and move in waves, like seaweed or a willow in the wind. Let your ribs, shoulders, and head go with the luscious motion. Enjoy this for several minutes.

Then gradually make the movement smaller and smaller. Continue to let your head just bobble on top as you come closer to center. What sense lets you know where center is? See how subtle the undulation can be—almost as delicate as a thought. Melt inside with these delectable sensations.

The Sweetness of Space

This movement meditation on flow is a natural extension of any of the other meditations described here. Explore it first in a relaxed sitting position; later you can try it standing. Remember that there is no wrong way to do this.

Settle in, taking as much time as you want. Then become aware of how the space wraps all around your body in a loving embrace. Feel the gentle touch of the air on your skin—on your cheeks, arms, eyelids, throat. Enjoy its sweet caress.

When you are ready, begin "Floating Hands." Keeping your fingers and elbows softly relaxed, allow your hands to rise slowly into the space, as if they are being magnetized upward, until they float in front of you. Imagine that the texture of the space is viscous and supportive, like an ocean of honey.

Begin to move your hands and fingers very slowly and sensitively. Explore the sensations of buoyancy and the luscious texture of the air. Feel its imaginary thickness or lightness, the quality of the touch. As you move, shift your attention back and forth between being active and being receptive. Gently stroke and tickle the air. Then pause and receive its touch. Imagine that the space gently tickles, strokes, and nudges you.

Give yourself an eternity to soak up the sweetness of this contact. Your hands may become so responsive that they begin to subtly drift of their own accord, as though lovingly moved by invisible currents around you. Surrender to this dance.

❧ REFLECTIONS

- What happens in your body when you allow compassion in? What sensations do you notice? What emotions? What insights about yourself?
- How has your awareness of space changed? Your sense of flow?
- These new thoughts, emotions, and sensations take some getting used to; that's why it's called meditation *practice*. You are developing "inner muscles" for the compassion that is fundamental to your health and happiness.

✌ SECRET #5
DWELL IN YOUR INNER SANCTUARY

Something's not right. I feel off.
Am I ever looking forward to this meditation, to check into what's going on.
If only I had a cave somewhere to retreat to . . .
To lick my wounds, even though I don't know what they are!
I'll create an inner cave and just . . . breathe . . .

My chest is so . . . tight, as though something is tugging on my heart.
Hmm, not exactly sadness . . .
Disheartened . . . oh, I'm . . . disheartened.

So much effort . . . I really do try to give my all.
I give and give, but sometimes it just doesn't seem enough.
I know this is just a mood, but I could just . . . weep.
My heart, my heart is . . . hungry! Maybe I'm just depleted.
Okay, hungry heart, let me feed you with the breath.
I'll focus on the inhalation, really take it in. I could use some inspiration . . .

"I receive breath."
Ah, soft movement of the breath coming in, that's it.
A little shallow, but easy does it, no forcing. Exhale.
Another inhalation, umm, a little deeper.
"I receive life." Yes, then just let the exhalation go.
Inhale: "I receive love."
Ah, my chest is beginning to soften a little.
A trickle of love flows in. . . . A trickle of tears flows out.

"I receive breath . . . I receive life . . . I receive love."
Yes, yes. I feel it now. Life is flowing into me, filling me, nourishing me.
Tender touch of the breath in and out—melting, softening . . .

I receive and release, over and over again.
How generous this movement of breath . . . how gentle . . .
I don't have to do anything—just be here with it, with myself.
"I receive life. I receive love . . ."
Ah, let me dwell inside this cave of the heart, forever!

ex ex ex

GIVE YOURSELF SPACE

Women are empathetic creatures. We are sensitive to pain, tension, and all that is unresolved in the world. We carry this collective tension in our bodies and psyches.

If you do not have sanctuary from the world, you cannot metabolize all the subtle feelings you have for other people and the burden of emotion you carry for others. The de-stressing process in meditation helps to unburden your heart. This frees up a tremendous amount of psychic energy, transmuting tension into creativity and love.

In the outer world a sanctuary is a sacred place, such as a temple, a mosque, or a church. Sanctuaries are also established to protect wildlife, as in bird sanctuaries, where hunting is prohibited. The word *sanctuary* comes from a Latin root meaning "to make sacred" or "to consecrate." A magic circle is drawn about the place, and all within it are under the protection of God.

In daily life a sanctuary is a place where you can rest and be yourself. You are safe from attack and from being hunted. You can relax totally, and you are safe to unwind, to let go, to let your guard down. Such rest can feel sacred, profoundly nourishing and healing. A time of sanctuary renews you and lets you emerge into the world stronger.

To go deep in meditation, you need to be able to create a sanctuary for yourself. That means giving yourself a space that is yours, even if only temporarily, and a time that is yours, even if it's only a moment. Your sanctuary may be your garden, or the bathtub, or your bedroom, or the sofa in the living room. That space becomes your sanctuary because you make it so.

The act of giving yourself space for meditation can feel quite assertive—you may have to push other things aside, close the door, say no to this demand or that one. Put a "Go Away" or "Do Not Disturb

Meditation" sign on the door and unplug the phone or turn the ringer off. In so doing, you erect a protective boundary so that you will not have to think about being invaded or interrupted.

Taking space is also intimate, daring, and courageous. You are giving yourself the privacy to commune with the depths of your being. You are setting up the situation so that you can reconnect with your quiet inner self. When there is sanctuary, you can drift into the space between things. Meditation is a "liminal" state: it happens at the threshold between the inner world and the outer world. You touch the sheer membrane between conscious and unconscious, between dream and reality, and penetrate beneath the surface to sense the creative stirrings of your soul.

Creating sanctuary can be as simple or as elaborate as you choose. You may want to have a special place in your home to meditate. Some women create beautiful altars with symbolic objects, photos of their family, a vase of flowers. Prayer can create a sanctuary, and for some people prayer is the way to begin. Invoke something greater than yourself: a healing presence, a higher power, the divine. You might light a candle or burn incense that you enjoy. For some women, cleaning around the meditation place creates the refuge; for others, dancing around it is what creates the refuge. And then there are those women who just plunk down with no fuss at all—instant sanctuary.

If for some reason it is not practical to make a sanctuary at home, consider finding a church, a garden, or an outdoor spot you can use.

Give Yourself Time

You only need half an hour, but make it uninterrupted, unrushed, and unhurried. Allow five minutes at the end to just sit there. Schedule enough time so that you won't have to rush off somewhere. A full practice would be to meditate for twenty minutes in the morning before breakfast and again in the afternoon or evening before dinner. It takes a while to settle in and get present before you start doing a technique. I usually sit for five minutes just drinking my tea. The reason for timing the meditation part is that it is a state of such deep rest that you want to take it in appropriate doses. You want to get used to such a state very gradually, over a period of months. It is quite intense to walk down the street with your senses wide open, totally relaxed inside. If you meditate too much too soon, you may become overly sensitive or languid during your activities.

The most common complaint of the general population is that there is not enough time in the day. Who has time to meditate? But here's one of those paradoxes: meditation can actually give you time. As you learn through meditation to stay with your own rhythms, you gain the clarity and presence of mind needed to organize your day. Your priorities fall into place, and with a more relaxed attitude, you gain a sense of having even more time and space for what is truly important.

WOMEN AND STRESS

We all long for healthy balance in our lives. Everyone knows that stress is a prime factor in many medical conditions. Too much stress takes us out of pleasure. Some stress is beneficial, and even pleasurable; optimal levels give us just the right degree of stimulation, and the excitement of a full and meaningful life can even strengthen the immune response. It's excessive and prolonged strain that causes problems.

At the biological level it is the parasympathetic nervous system, which gives us the rest-and-restore mode, that keeps our hearts and blood vessels open, while the sympathetic nervous system, the fight-or-flight part, constricts the heart and blood vessels, keeping them toned. Every blood vessel in the body is filigreed with both nerve systems because we need both modes to live fully. Finding the equilibrium between rest and action, between letting go and going for it, is our contemporary challenge. In general, the mental and physical texture of daily life is too fast, dense, and pressured, so we need to make a conscious effort to cultivate the opposite tones.

Medical research is turning up some very significant information on how female biology differs from male biology. Most studies have been done on male subjects, and their conclusions generalized from men's bodies (just as in the meditation field!). Fortunately, this situation is finally beginning to change. A recent report suggests that females are less likely to react to stress with the fight-or-flight response typical of males and more likely to "tend and befriend"—that is, to find ways to nurture and seek the support of others. The study finds that this response happens in both humans and animals and is based on hormonal differences between the sexes. Aggression is an important energy for women to have access to when necessary. But in the face of everyday stress we can also nurture each other and ourselves, creating a network of supportive relationships.

Many of the mental stressors that everyone contends with are not likely to go away. We are a headstrong society. Managing information overload, keeping up with technology, sitting at the computer for long hours each day, constantly strategizing to maintain status or get ahead—these are the necessities of modern life. The electronic bombardment itself toys with our nervous systems. Even when exercising, people are often not really in their bodies at all as they simultaneously read, watch TV, or listen to music through headsets. But being "in our heads" takes a serious toll, and the consequent lack of relaxation and deep pleasure is especially hazardous to women. Chronic, persistent stress weakens the immune system and plays a role in the development of heart disease. Stress also powerfully affects our mental well-being. Women's bodies are wonderfully sensitive, and our nervous systems can easily become overwhelmed. In addition, there is evidence that excessive head-centered attention may disrupt the female glandular system and hormonal balance, with far-reaching consequences to our general health.

Each woman must come to terms with this conundrum in her own way. Modern society is unlikely to change, but there are many effective measures we can take to care for ourselves. Scientists consistently recommend certain antidotes for women: exercise, expression, relaxation, and self-exploration. We couldn't agree more.

You need exercise that you can enjoy and look forward to, not activity that is just an onerous discipline. Find whatever calls you forth—walking, dance, yoga, swimming, martial arts. Challenge the temptation to make an object of your body, to look at it as a lump of flesh that you must whip into shape. The element of pleasure is extremely important, and if you can find exercise that pleases your soul, all the better. Dance has the added benefit of poetic and emotional expressiveness. Some sports also facilitate a kind of expression. Women who engage in aggressive exercise like kick-boxing have been shown to experience less depression and stronger immune systems. The kick-butt attitude gives them a sense of power and control over their lives. In addition to dynamic forms that increase circulation, we recommend (no, insist!) that you include stretching to maintain flexibility and fluidity. Staying supple is especially crucial as the years go by; aging tends to dry us out and make us rigid—mentally and physically. This is preventable, so don't forget to lengthen and soften those muscles.

As for relaxation, self-exploration, and expression, the approach to meditation that we are suggesting addresses all three. Finding meditations that work for you is the ultimate in self-care and self-awareness. Nothing relaxes like the pleasure of meditation, which puts you in touch with your inner world. In that safety you can discover and support whatever needs to be expressed and embodied in your life.

GIVING AND RECEIVING

The movement of giving and receiving is the basic circulation of life energy, and this movement is vital to every human being. In every breath we exercise the ability to receive life, to draw in the love that we need, as well as the ability to release, to express, to give. The full flow of inhaling and exhaling is a sign of health, an intimate and immediate connection to the source of life.

Most of us experience an inhibition in that full circulation, usually stemming from the conditions of early childhood when some expression, some outflow of our emotion, was not accepted. Or maybe it was not safe to relax and receive. Somehow our flow was interrupted consistently enough that we learned to accommodate, to hold back the energy, in order to feel safe and accepted—and doing so became a habit.

You may literally hold your breath. This habit in turn affects how you encounter the world around you—perhaps with a hidden sense of fear or isolation. When you become conscious of the holding pattern, you can begin to soften. The obstruction may manifest in physical discomfort or tension. Consider this a signal to yourself to let go, to receive, or to express.

To receive the flow of love is such a fundamental requirement that to recognize how you have not received it can bring up sorrow. To give love is an equally basic requirement, and sometimes the greater sorrow is in seeing how you have held back the flow of your love for others. The honesty of revealing these underlying patterns brings tremendous

∾ MEDITATION ON GIVING AND RECEIVING

Every breath is an effortless act of giving and receiving. When we make this movement conscious, we weave ourselves into greater connection with the source of life, with our loved ones, and with all of humanity.

Step 1

Take some time to become present. When you have settled in, bring your attention to your breathing. After a minute or so, begin to focus on the intake of breath. To inhale is literally "inspiration." Meditate with these phrases: *I receive breath. I receive life. I receive love.* With each inhalation say one of the phrases with your inner voice. Speak directly to yourself and breathe in the quality those words evoke for you. Spend as long as you like exploring this receptive state.

Step 2

Bring your attention to the exhalation. You can choose to do this in the same meditation or on some other day, whenever you want to augment the sense of flowing out toward the world. In the same way, begin to focus on the outflow of the breath. Repeat these words inside yourself: *I give breath. I give life. I give love.* Let the breath stream out with each phrase and imbue the exhalation with whatever meaning it has for you. Send that quality forth with each exhalation—to God, to the world, to someone you care about.

Step 3

Explore taking the feelings into movement. Begin with "Floating Hands." Draw your hands inward toward your face, heart, or belly as you say, "I receive breath. I receive life. I receive love." Move your hands outward as you say, "I give breath. I give life. I give love." This is your spontaneous dance of giving and receiving.

This meditation can elicit a range of emotion as you become more aware of your longings—what you have within you to give as well as what you need. Let it open your heart to the intimacy you desire.

relief but initially can be so uncomfortable that you may stop meditating. Don't cheat yourself of this transformative gift.

In your meditation, explore the spacious movement of giving and receiving. Release into all the love you want to give, and all you can receive. You'll feel a gentle internal stretch, a fuller breath as you open to life. This simple meditation, an enduring teaching on intimacy and satisfaction, can last you a lifetime.

CREATE SAFETY FOR YOURSELF

Safety is fundamental in any kind of inner work. The processes of heal-ing are natural, but they happen best when we feel safe. If we do not feel safe, healing will wait, politely, until we are. Meditations that call forth a feeling of safety build a strong container for healing.

The instinct for sanctuary can be observed throughout the animal kingdom, both wild and domestic. Most animals seek out safe shelter to hide, to groom, to rest—inside a cave, under a bush, in a corner behind the couch. Our animal friends are great mentors on relaxation, safety, and retreat. They know how to take care of themselves.

One element of feeling safe is knowing that you do not have to act on what you think. Remind yourself from time to time to accept all your thoughts:

- I am not going to be judged for what I think during meditation.
- I am not accountable for the content.
- I do not need to edit or censor.
- It is my brain doing its work.
- I do not need to interfere.
- This kind of thing goes on all the time in sleep and dreams when I am not awake (and able to interfere).

& THE REDWOOD REFUGE

This meditation illustrates how individual and nonliteral the image of sanctuary can be. Lillian discovered it in a session while going through a torturous separation from a man she loved. Wrenched in body and heart, she craved a place beyond the pain where she could rest and find solace and strength. It began with a suggestion to lie on her back and feel herself carried by the ground.

"I am floating on my back inside of a redwood tree. I am safe within the tree, alone and private. My arms and legs are spread out, so I am like a five-pointed star, floating and warm within the safety of the tree."

Lillian reported: "This meditation was an amazing healing, very visual and vis-ceral for me. I used to go there all the time, and I would instantly feel fine. All the pain was gone. It couldn't touch me. Resting in my inner sanctuary gave me the clar-ity I needed to find my way through the outer situation."

Safety Always Leads to De-stressing

Safety leads to a release of the tensions you carry around. This is the paradoxical nature of meditation: you are safe to notice how unsafe you have felt. Relaxation leads to the release of muscular tension, which in turn leads you to review what you've been tense about. This process may look on the surface like worrying but is actually your brain freeing itself up from the tyranny of the past and getting ready for action. Unless you realize this, you may judge yourself when such experiences come up.

The pleasure and dilation of meditation creates more space in which to witness your thoughts and impulses. It is important to accept whatever comes up, even the uncomfortable feelings. There can be falling sensations as you let go, or a literal sense of darkness as you relax. These sensations can be scary to some people, so they resist. Remember that forbidden, fearful, lustful, or violent thoughts are part of your internal housekeeping. We can judge and repress a thought in milliseconds, so make sure that you create enough safety to tolerate the process.

If you are alive, there is no way to avoid tension; it's a normal consequence of interaction with the world. In the course of a day, we are constantly responding to our environment, both consciously and unconsciously. Much of the time we have to hold it all together and can't afford to acknowledge, much less indulge, these myriad reactions: irritation, fatigue, disappointment, fear, worry, shame. Those thousands of intricate little responses wriggle around in our nervous system with no place to go. When we have no time or place to assimilate them, they become embedded as habitual reactions to the world. We may even mistake our response to the stress for our true nature. For our sanity and our health, we absolutely require a release.

All these unconscious responses are Pavlovian conditioning: just thinking about that deadline, your boss, a difficult situation, gets you stressed. Even a tone of voice can seem like an attack (very common in intimate relationships!). The body doesn't like performing under stress, because tension does not serve the body's optimum functioning. Meditation is a deconditioning; the outer event and the response are decoupled. You no longer react mechanically, and after meditation you are free to make up a new response.

What goes on instinctively when you engage your senses in meditation is analogous to a vaccination against stress. When your body is presented with a weakened form of a virus, the invader is recognized and the body learns to take appropriate measures. Meditation builds up your ability to deal with stress without getting infected. It brings you moments of indolent peacefulness, then draws you into reviewing the situations that have made you tense, grated on your nerves, made you flinch or overreact. You witness everything in slow motion. Your body tends to take apart all the sounds and images: how you went into emergency mode, how you got alarmed. As you reexperience fragments of the stressors, your body practices staying relaxed and at ease. In this way it learns how to maintain its integrity when the stress recurs.

Fear

Unprocessed fear is a common pattern held in the body that surfaces when people begin to meditate. Chronic fear is physiologically unnatural. During meditation, when you are relaxed and safe, you can face your fears by allowing them to rise to the surface to be examined.

When we submit to the process of de-stressing, uncomfortable as it is, we reclaim the world for ourselves and reclaim our intuition. Fear is just for the moment, for emergencies. In emergency situations, the instinctive "fight or flight" response kicks in, supplying the body with adrenaline and other stress hormones so that we can defend ourselves. But if we habitually act as if there is an emergency when there is not, the stress persists, those hormones don't get processed, and they end up poisoning our bodies—and our perception of the world. Cultivating safety in meditation gives you a focus to which you can return, again and again, so that the fear can wash out of your system.

Anxiety

Anxiety is a common complaint of women, exacerbated by our hormones, not to mention our busyness. Both can make us feel overwhelmed, without resources. "I can't handle it!" we cry. We are consumed with worries: "What if . . . ?" Anxiety and worry arise from the mental evaluation of a situation. When we encounter something challenging, we unconsciously determine its size (is it bigger than I am?), whether it is a threat, and whether we can deal with it. Worry is not a problem when we have access to our pleasure and sense of power. But sometimes these resources seem totally out of reach.

🙝 TIPS FOR RELIEVING ANXIETY

Try "Thumbs Up," a simple exercise from *jin shin jyutsu* that helps to alleviate worry and anxiety. Hold your thumb with the other hand for a few minutes. Change hands when you want. That's it. You can do this almost anywhere. It's a little like sucking your thumb, very comforting and balancing.

It also helps to:

- Take hot baths
- Drink soothing teas
- Get more sleep
- Find more comfort
- Have more orgasms
- Be massaged
- Receive acupuncture
- Reduce or eliminate caffeine and sugar
- Add B vitamins, calcium, and other nutrients to your diet
- Take "Calms Forte" (a homeopathic remedy)
- Simplify, simplify, simplify—any way possible

Even though much of meditation is thinking, and much of thinking is worry, meditating is profoundly different from obsessing. You are inviting your nervous system to break up that pattern by the interaction between the focus and the spontaneous movement of attention. You are not just reviewing your life; you are in a different state that gives you resources and presents new options. By giving yourself a special time to let any thought come, to release control and give the brain free rein, you are giving yourself what you need. After meditation your mind feels clear and you're ready for life. Women report that they don't even remember what they were worrying about!

In terms of energy, anxiety is a mental state with a physical correlation: congestion in the head. Energy needs to flow down out of the head to the lower body, down through the belly, legs, and feet. Anxiety is a clue that earth energy is calling you, that you need to restore your sense of containment and ground (see "Secret #9: Rest in Simplicity"). You may first need to exaggerate the jagged, jittery sensations in movement, tensing and releasing your muscles until you become more relaxed.

Then meditate and soften your thoughts, soften your face, soften your chest, soften your belly. Imagine a flow of energy down from your forehead all the way to your feet.

ILLNESS AS SANCTUARY

Having time off from all your obligations is a necessity, though not often recognized as such, so the need for retreat, for privacy and rest, is sometimes provided by default through illness. The downside to living in such an "advanced" civilization is that we are overly identified with work, productivity, and action. Some people refuse to take time out and override their very real need to rest until it escalates and they absolutely must stop in their tracks. Getting sick is a culturally legitimate excuse to say no to what people expect. Who can question that you deserve time to yourself? Illness provides us with the one time it's okay to give over, to let down completely, to be a bump in the bed, or to do whatever is necessary to heal and regenerate. If you are ill, make the most of the situation; do it up, royally. Pamper yourself, or get someone else to pamper you.

In some families (and some New Age circles), getting sick is a source of shame: "You've been thinking the wrong thoughts." In others, illness is a way to have your own neediness recognized, to get relief from being the caretaker, the hard worker, the go-getter. Sickness may seem like the only way out of unpleasant circumstances for some women. A worthy inquiry, before you actually get sick, is to ask, "What secret fulfillment would I gain from illness?" Then why not give that to yourself more directly?

Telling the truth about what you really want and need is a challenge. It can be tempting to say, "You know, I'm not feeling very well," when the truth is that you simply do not want to do something, do not want to be with someone, or crave time alone for whatever reason.

Meditation is preemptive. You take the radical step of giving yourself the time and space you require.

SILENCE

Many people, when they sit to meditate, recognize an intense craving for silence. Our lives are so complex; there is so much stimulation, so much information, so many demands, so much noise! This assault on the senses takes a lot out of us. We truly need a respite from the overload, but it's not easily achieved. Meditation gives us the space and time to disengage from the onslaught and can lead us into a lusciously serene silence and solitude.

When you get quiet, you may notice how tired you are of talking. We expend a tremendous amount of energy in speaking—it just leaks right out through our mouths! Sometimes I crave my own silence as much as I crave food or sleep; I simply cannot utter another word. To give in to that craving is luxuriously restful and extremely satisfying. Take a few hours or even a day in silence. Start with whatever amount of time you can manage; being silent is especially regenerative at the very beginning or end of the day. Warn your friends and family that you won't be available (one of those taboos you may need to break). Let someone else take care of the kids. From the time you get up until sunset, if possible, don't speak. Turn the phone ringer off. Meditate a few times. There is alchemy in containing your energy. Just making the decision to be silent for a while evokes power, and a blanket of shimmering silence will descend upon you like a silk robe that you wear throughout the day.

Silence is not just absence of sound but a rich and vibrant harmony that seems to underlie and support all other vibration. Musicians are aware of the power of silence, the space between the notes, as the fertile ground from which all music emerges and to which it returns. When you meditate, you are like a fine instrument in the hands of the cosmic tuner: your nervous system is gently and skillfully brought into accord with the healing music of the universe.

Mantras and inner sounds can function like a tuning fork. You think of a sound, let it fade away, and as your senses follow it into the silence you become more attuned and harmonized.

Inner Silence and Outer Noise

Outer noises often intrude on our sanctuary. Birds can be incredibly noisy, motors hum in the distance or up close, jets fly overhead, people talk, doors open and shut, waves break on the shore.

There is a very straightforward way to deal with noise—don't even have an opinion about it. Don't let yourself care if the sounds are there or not—as you would if you were reading escape fiction in a coffee shop or airport. Do what you can to give yourself some protection from the noise, but other than that, don't fuss.

When a new sound comes to your attention, what is the easiest thing to do? Simply listen without resistance, without thinking you should be concentrating against the noise. Your attention will follow the sound and soon lose interest. This is the fundamental attitude to cultivate about noises, and this suggestion will make your path in meditation much easier.

After you get a foundation in simplicity about noise, you can evolve your play further:

- *Transparency:* You tolerate the experience of sound passing right through you, enlivening your nerves for a moment. Sound is a wave, after all.

- *Shock:* The sound wakes you up, startles you, and you can welcome the awakening. The shock can be a real surprise because sometimes in meditation you are very deep in silence.

- *Rebound into silence:* Sometimes a sound can make you aware of how silent the space around you was and, as the sound passes, *still is.* The sound carries you into the silence.

- *Match the sound:* If there is an irritating sound from outside that would ordinarily drive you nuts, sometimes you can counter it with a similar vibration inside. Use the same capacity you have to play a song in your head, and play that same sound in your head that you are hearing outside.

For example, one morning I was sitting on the sofa meditating, with the sliding glass door onto the lawn open. The gardener came by with his leaf blower and was blowing leaves from one side of the patio to the other, then back again. As its loud, searing sound entered my nervous system, I felt a shock of irritation (detestable machines, one of my pet peeves). But then I realized that it was only a sound, a kind of strange music, so I began to hum the same tone inside myself, like a mantra: *jzzzjjzzz.* Immediately I felt relieved and oddly empowered, and even started to laugh. The leaf blower sound couldn't get to me; I was meeting the noise with an equal frequency and sending it out of my body as

---

❧ THE GODDESS IN MY LIVING ROOM

This is a meditation from Cherise, a singer and mother of a four-year-old daughter. Sometimes she gets only five minutes of solitude, but those precious moments infuse her day.

"In the mornings I sit on the sofa in my living room and arrange pillows around me, surrounding me, so I am simultaneously surrounded, cuddled, and enthroned. I am the goddess of the living room.

"I know my daughter is going to wake up in a few minutes, but I don't have to pick anything up, and the light is perfect.

"For these few minutes I am nurtured. I breathe in the elixir of creation. I drink the mother's milk of the vast spaciousness extending in all directions, and I let the mystery of breath massage me and care for me. I am filled to overflowing with the essence of the feminine, so I have it to give away and for myself as well.

"Then my daughter will come out and flitter around me like a little bug, and I will engage with her, and miraculously, it will not feel chaotic. I can be centered and in some kind of mobile peacefulness that is able to keep up with her. This is an everyday miracle. I can be rested and relaxed and able to play and then go to work and come back and engage with her again."

---

a vibratory song. It was "The Leaf Blower Duet." My nerves had been a bit wrought up anyway—this was happening at the end of a hard week—so the hum that I invented matched my internal buzz and ended up providing an unexpected balm. Nevertheless, when the gardener left, I was quite pleased.

All these ways of being with outside noises are also ways of welcoming the world and feeling snug in your sanctuary.

Some meditators get into a habit of resenting outside noises, but this attitude can be fatal to your meditation. Pull that weed right away; it can take over your garden. If you resent outside noise, you are making the world wrong for existing and moving. You have set yourself against the movement of life. The resentment is probably based on pain, the pain of the sound hitting your raw nerves, and the cure is probably to let the ease and the rest of your sanctuary time heal those nerves.

❧

IN DEFENSE OF LAZINESS

Often when people get the inner silence they crave, they judge it as laziness, sleepiness, indolence, weakness, or depression. Often people spend years trapped in this mind-set, sabotaging their own inner peace.

Many other cultures know how to relax and move at a much slower pace; they live in a flowing sense of time, an eternal now. Americans are very gung-ho, with a lot of creative energy and enthusiasm. Beneath our manic energy lie a Puritan heritage and a work ethic that never rests. We tend to abhor silence and emptiness; space and time must always be filled. Our culture is so obviously afflicted with this surfeit of doing and poverty of being that it is even endearing in a pathetic sort of way. But just knowing that what you're up against is culturally relative can give you freedom of choice.

Scientifically speaking, when you meditate, you are resting more deeply than in sleep. The feeling is luxuriously lazy. If you find resistance to such relaxation, be aware that you literally need to feel through this reaction and face your fear of laziness. Insecurity comes up sometimes from simply letting yourself be.

Many women admit to difficulty in allowing themselves rest, with supermoms at the top of the list. Men seem to find it easier to work hard and then let down and play. Because women are used to self-sacrifice and are trained to care for other people's needs, they tend to feel guilty taking time for themselves. How much of this is necessity, and how much is conditioning? Try this little experiment: what happens when you consider these statements?

I don't have time for myself.
I do have time for myself.
What would it be like if I had more time for myself?

The judgment against down time is also a family pattern. If not interfered with, most children will naturally meditate—by staring at the ceiling or visually tracing the lines on the wall. If it wasn't safe for you to "space out" this way in your own childhood, you may still expect attack or hear the adult voices from long ago telling you to get to work, to be sociable, to help out. "What are you doing? Get up. Be productive. You're wasting your time!" When parents come barging in on you, fear is created. A mother can often intuit what her child is doing in the next room. If she is fraught with tension herself, her nerves may tingle with oversensitivity. When there's a shift of attention in the child, a concentration or relaxation (masturbation is a prime example), the mother feels it. This is the dark side of intuition—an invasion of personal privacy.

If there is depression in the family system, just sitting still may evoke the fear of mental illness. Constant chatter and activity may cloak a silent dread—that some secret might be told, or someone might go nuts—some elephant in the living room that nobody will admit.

The story of Nora, a therapist in her sixties, reveals how deep the taboo against resting can be. Her family structure was riddled with depression and denial, a manic mother and a sibling suicide. After decades of inner work and much improvement, she is still haunted by anxiety when she has the chance to rest. Such patterns are deeply ingrained, and Nora may always need to counter this pattern with conscious body wisdom, an understanding she now imparts to her patients. We all have these life challenges, places in us that require special care. They are the wounds that can become our teaching gifts.

When you do have the space to rest, what you crave comes to your attention. This rattles your status quo; you can expect that. Many of the cravings that we awaken to in meditation are not new. Meditation gives you the resources to face them. Allow yourself to explore your cravings—for example, the feelings you had as a ten-year-old that had to be denied because conditions were not safe. You put them off for later, postponed them so that you could get on with your life. They got stuck in your attic, under a rug, or in a closet. When you give in to the cravings, parallel feelings come up, perhaps on several tracks simultaneously. You feel the aftereffects of having denied your needs and desires. You also feel the fear of them actually being fulfilled.

Learn to be lazy, consciously. Meditation is "much ado about nothing," as close to doing nothing as you can get. This rest takes getting used to, but it is a favor to yourself that you'll never regret. The famous meditators of the ages were actually diligent couch potatoes, watching the inner screen and changing the channel from the astral frequency to transcendental bliss. So call it "sacred laziness." The lazier you are for concentrated periods, the more you can recharge and then approach your life creatively with renewed balance and vigor.

THE IMPORTANCE OF TRANSITIONS

Transitions before and after significant events deserve deliberate attention. They are formative opportunities to make new choices about your life.

When transitional time is not honored, the nervous system can be very disrupted. Maybe you've experienced how jarring it is, for example, after a moving performance or film if the lights come up too fast. The audience claps obediently or gets up right away. People go on automatic, and the moment passes as if nothing had happened. The rich atmosphere is dispelled, and there is no time taken to digest the emotional impact of the event.

At the end of most yoga classes there is a five-minute period of *Savasana,* or "Corpse Pose," in which you lie on your back and completely let go. Not only is this a profound mini-meditation, but it gives your whole system a chance to integrate the shifts your body has made. Then, when you gradually bring movement back into your body, you experience a rebirth to the world. Give yourself this same period of transition after meditation.

Be very gradual and aware as you emerge from your sanctuary. This is especially important after a long meditation, retreat, or vacation, when your nervous system has had a chance to come into balance. When you reenter the world at large, you are likely to observe more objectively the compulsive pace and fragmentation around you. You feel the seduction of your ordinary habits of reaction. But this is a special chance to see through these patterns and to make new choices about how you want to live. Give yourself time to make that adjustment and to create the texture of life that you crave.

❧ EXPLORATIONS

- When and how do you give yourself space? (for example, reading, being alone, taking a walk, taking a bath)

- When do you take space? In other words, when do you fill up the space with your own energy? (for example, cleaning, arranging or decorating a room, singing, praying)

- When you were little, how did you space out? What natural meditations did you do? For example, did you stare at the pattern of

> ✇ **WARM-UP: CREATE YOUR INNER SANCTUARY**
>
> A sanctuary gives you a sense of boundaries, containment, safety, and solitude. Your inner sanctuary can be like a garden, a temple, an island, a mountain, a fort, a cave, or a cathedral. Occasionally I go to a distant galaxy to get away.
>
> What is your image of sanctuary? Let your imagination have free rein with this. Construct your internal sanctuary anywhere and in any way you desire. Decorate the imaginary space with your favorite colors, flowers, or icons; furnish your inner world exactly as you choose.
>
> Then place yourself inside the image, relax in its safety, and receive the particular qualities this sacred place provides. Stay there as long as you have time for, simply dwelling within. You can begin every meditation by establishing sanctuary in this way. Over time your image of sanctuary will probably change according to what you require. Let this be an ongoing process of discovery.

the wallpaper, curtains, or floor? Did you sit on a rock listening to the gurgle of a stream, lie on your back gazing at the stars, sit in a secret garden or under a favorite tree? How did your parents react when they found you being "lazy"?

- Cultivate the sense of safety. Explore places where you feel safe: the beach, the movie theater, a church or synagogue, the sofa, your favorite chair, under the covers, in the bath. Notice the subtle relaxation in your belly, chest, neck, and jaw as you dwell in safety.

- Make a simple prayer. Write it in your journal and learn it by heart.

✇ SKILL CIRCLE #5: HOW TO MEDITATE WITH A MANTRA

Sound is a handy focus for meditation because we use sound in spoken language as well as in internal thinking. Using a mantra tunes you in to the auditory quality of thinking. The murmuring of the mantra creates a subtle vibration in your nerves, a very refined vibratory massage. When we use sound as a focus in meditation, we can follow it right into the silence.

When you meditate, you'll become even more aware of fatigue from the noise you listen to every day. You'll notice the pain of your nerves as they shift gears. Even your own thoughts may seem too noisy. Watch out now: the craving for mental silence can lead to an attempt to block out thoughts. This is not helpful. Not only is this barrier impossible, but it succeeds only in putting you at war with yourself. Instead, learn to stay with the particular weird sensations as your nerves heal. Eventually you will shift from defended mode to relaxation, embracing the silence like an old and cherished friend.

Elemental Sound

The sounds of speech are useful not only for expressing ourselves in the outer world; they also take us into the inner world. You can begin by exploring your relationship with the vowels of your mother tongue. In English that is *a, e, i, o, u,* and sometimes *y.* Each region of the world has its own way of pronouncing a vowel, and those differences are interesting and charming. What you want to do in this exercise is to let yourself be intrigued by the sounds themselves and the way they resonate in your body. This sounds like child's play, and it is. There is a great deal of similarity between meditation and child's play.

Start by singing or humming the vowels in any way that occurs to you, at any volume, speed, or pitch. Just get a playful, exploratory expression going. Feel free to change the order after a while—*u-e-a,* for example. Change the pronunciation however you like, for each sound has a dozen or so different ways of being said. Your preferences are important and may change with the time of day, according to how tired or energetic you are, and according to whether the sound is external and audible or purely internal and audible only to the mind's ear.

Select two vowel sounds, *a-u, e-o,* or any combination you prefer in this instant. Say that sound over and over softly, in a kind of chant. Let the sound become quieter over the course of several minutes and simply enjoy the rhythm of the sound, the vibrations in your head and throat, the subtle movements of your tongue, and the flow of the breath. Your eyes can be open or closed, and you can go back and forth between open and closed.

At some point in the next several minutes let the softly audible chant become an internal chant. Let this transition happen in its own time, gradually.

When the chant becomes internal, it may change in various ways. Sometimes it continues as before and you are simply listening to the sound mentally. The chant can fluctuate in volume, from being loud and distinct in your inner hearing to being soft and faint. Then it may fade away, leaving you there listening to the silence, or to the absence of sound. Welcome this nothingness, or blank space, or "forgetting," and train yourself not to panic or to think you have failed when your mind goes silent. At some point there will probably be little interludes, little quiet spaces between sounds in which you can feel your body vibrating. Sometimes the sound will go in sync with your breath, sometimes not. One of the vowels may become extended indefinitely—for example, *o* may become *ooooooooooooo*.

As you listen inwardly to the sound or sounds in a restful way, you may notice relaxed feelings coming over you, alternating with thoughts about what time it is, what you have to do next, and any worries you have. Train yourself to welcome this process, then gently return to the vowels. Do not concentrate, even a little. If the vowels are interesting to you, you will enjoy playing with them. If you do not enjoy the sounds themselves, then don't do this exercise at this time. The amount of effort you use to pay attention to the vowels should be slightly less than you use to read—about the amount of effort your eyes make to glide across a page.

Use this simple exercise to cultivate your sense of preference for sound, and in particular to heighten your appreciation of how beautiful the vowels are. Give yourself the freedom to discover what you love about sound, both inner sound and thoughts, and the sounds we use in speech. You may discover that you love the space before speech when you are looking for an appropriate word or sound to express what you are feeling, or possibly the silence after speech, when you have said something. The essence of meditation is to discover, not impose.

After you become comfortable with the basic vowel sounds and familiar with how they affect your body, explore the sounds you associate with delight, pleasure, surprise, wonder, awe, and relief. These could be sounds such as *ahhhh, ohhhh, wow,* and *whew.* This exercise will help you to construct your own sound to use in meditation, or it may sensitize you so that you can pick one of the many great mantras used in the religions of the world, such as *Allelujah, Amen, OM,* or *AUM.*

Doing this elemental sound exercise is good preparation for using a mantra in meditation because you give yourself a chance to develop a sense of playfulness and leisure, which in turn leads to a deeper sense of safety and rest. Playfulness is the perfect antidote to trying too hard—a primary obstacle to meditating properly.

Taking Refuge in Sacred Names

The sacred names do not "belong" to any one group; no one owns God. At the same time there is absolutely no reason to change your religion or impose a theology on yourself in order to meditate.

You can choose a mantra from the names of the goddesses and gods of any of the sacred traditions of the world. Select a mantra based on the types of sound you long to hear. Sound can be soothing, harmonizing, and electrifying. Here are a few to memorize and explore:

- To surround yourself with the quality of compassion and mercy, chant the Chinese Kwan Yin mantra: *Na mo kwan shih yin pu sa.*

- To celebrate the Great Mother, chant the Hindu mantra: *Shri ma namah* (shree mah namah).

- To evoke the intensity of Kali energy, chant the Hindu mantra: *Hrim krim* (hreem kreem).

- To express devotion to the god Shiva, the male principle of creation, chant: *Om namah shivaya.*

- To express devotion to Shakti, the feminine principle of creation, chant: *Shrim shaktim* (shreem shakteem).

- To evoke transcendent consciousness, chant a Tibetan Buddhist mantra that means "the Jewel in the Lotus": *Om mane padme hum* (ohm mahnay padmay hoom).

- Make a mantra of the names of God: *Elohim. Allah. Yahweh.*

As described earlier, repeat the sound externally or internally and bathe yourself in its vibration. Then let the sound carry you effortlessly into silence. Return periodically to the mantra.

Selecting a name of God as a mantra is a very intimate affair. It may seem awesome, as well it is. However, we have found that people have good instincts for what they need in meditation, so choose the one that you love or that appeals to you in some way.

You may want to take refuge in the sanctuary of a cathedral, temple, mosque, church, or meditation center to feel out your relationship with a name of God as a mantra. You can also pray and ask to be led to the perfect mantra for now. Mantras are private, and you don't need to tell anyone what you use.

Keep in mind that your mantra may change in a few years. Months are needed to really get used to a mantra. Feel free to explore and play, and stay with the ones you like.

Chanting

Another advantage of using sound as a focus is that your voice is employed. Let your voice be heard by chanting your favorite sounds.

Take a sound you crave and chant it repeatedly. Or use a hymn, poem, prayer, or song and sing it out, softly, loudly, reverently, wildly. Let the universe hear you! When the chant subsides, bask in the resonance within your body and the rich silence that remains.

Taking Sanctuary in Prayer

THE SALUTE TO THE DIVINE MOTHER

The Divine Mother dwells within me.
She shines through all of my senses.
Without Her, no sights could be seen, no sounds could be heard, no
*   words spoken.*
Although She shines through all of the senses, She cannot be grasped
*   by them.*
Although She enjoys all natural qualities, She remains beyond them and
*   is their witness.*
The Divine Mother dwells within me.
Shri ma namah.

The prayers of the world religions are an immense source of comfort, protection, and peace. Consider, for example, the Ninety-first Psalm of David. Such a prayer is almost a living being. The psalm has been cher-

ished by so many people over thousands of years that when you say it
you may feel that you are in an immense cathedral.

PSALM 91

He that dwelleth in the secret place of the most High
Shall abide under the shadow of the Almighty.
I will say of the LORD, He is my refuge and my fortress: my God; in Him
    will I trust.
Surely He shall deliver thee from the snare of the fowler, and from the
    noisome pestilence.
He shall cover thee with His feathers, and under His wings shalt thou trust:
His truth shall be thy shield and buckler.
Thou shalt not be afraid for the terror by night; nor for the arrow that
    flieth by day . . .

Learn these prayers by heart, so that the words just roll through your
awareness without any effort. This may take a month or so. Make friends
with each of the words and each of the images they call to mind. Spend a
few minutes daily with the prayer. After you know the prayer intimately,
even starting it, you are inside of its energy. The whole feeling tone of the
prayer is there in every word. You can rest in the prayer at the beginning
of your meditation to help create the feeling of sanctuary for yourself.

Music as Prayer Another way to take refuge in prayer is to listen to
Bach or any of the other great composers who have set prayers to
music. Writing religious music was how the composers made their living. Even if you aren't religious, you may be converted when you hear
an *Allelujah* chorus, or *The Passion of Saint Matthew*, or a requiem. If you
truly listen to this music, its devastating beauty will melt you and transform you. Also, the singers sound marvelous vowels of whatever language they are singing—Italian, German, English, Latin, French, or
Spanish.

Hunting for the music that speaks to your inmost heart is a very
worthwhile adventure. If you ask around, you will find allies in surprising places. Music is a universal language, and people with whom you
otherwise might have nothing to discuss can tell you of great performances they have heard live or on recordings.

There are many flavors of prayer, and when sung, each singer or composer brings a wholly new quality to it. The "color" that a particular singer brings to a prayer or hymn may resonate in your inner being as no other performance does. This experience opens a door in your heart. As you remember listening to the song, the remembered resonance gives you access to that level of feeling.

Sometimes when I am meditating the entire time is taken up in listening to music internally, savoring some incredible crescendo of feeling attained in a symphony. Symphonic music, one of the great accomplishments of humanity, can provide a wealth of blessing to everyone who meditates.

❧ MEDITATIONS

The Sanctuary of Your Personal Space

Seated comfortably, rest your hands in your lap and turn your palms to face each other. Take a few easy breaths, then gently become curious about the sensations in your palms. Explore moving your palms up and down, toward each other and away, in toward the body and away from it. Let your hands be very relaxed and loose, and still facing each other. You may have tiny sensations in your hands, pleasant feelings of warmth or tingling. Explore in this way for two or three minutes.

Tiny movements and slow motions of the hands can feel both very intense and unusually soothing. You probably have had few opportunities, in your entire life, to explore very slow motions, so be patient with yourself as you experiment.

Turn your hands outward and explore the space around your body within arm's reach. There is an egg-shaped zone around the body— your personal space. As a human animal, you can sense this zone. This is the space that you invite people into when you like them, and that you want them to stay out of if you don't. Your hands may tingle, or you may sense magnetism or some other sensation. Many people can sense their own aura, the magnetic energy rotating around the body, with no training at all. Their senses are capable of it, but they have never used them in this quiet way.

Make up your own hand dance, flowing gestures of the arms and hands that caress the inside of your aura or egg. Follow your sense of pleasure and wonder. As a basic vocabulary of movement to work with, you may explore these moves:

Gather your hands in toward your heart and rest them there for a heartbeat or two. Let them float outward as far as is comfortable, then sweep them around to either side. "From the core of my being, from my heart, a stream of love goes forth to surround me."

Rest your hands on the top of your head for a moment, then turn your palms to face upward, toward the sky. Let them flow upward as far as you can reach. "From the crown of my being I am related to the heavens." There are several chakras, or energy centers, above the head, and you may sense them as stars or radiant points of light.

Rest your hands in the lower part of your belly, and then gently allow them to glide outward. "From my belly, my womb, I am related to the generative powers of the earth, all the green growing things, and all the creativity of nature."

Let your hands rest between your legs, with your palms down toward the center of the earth. Notice that gravity pulls on your entire body, your arms, and your hands, and that the direction of gravity is always inward toward the center. Your body always knows exactly where the core of the earth is. As your hands are resting there, simply be aware of the relationship of your body and the earth. Half a minute of this may seem like a long, long time. Let your hands sweep slowly around your legs, as if painting a circle on the ground around you.

After making friends with the space around you, your aura, you may find that simply *beginning* one of these moves gives you a feeling of sanctuary within seconds, wherever you are.

Hum into Your Heart

Give yourself plenty of time to settle in. Then rest your hand on your breastbone near the heart and simply feel that contact for several breaths.

Start with a low hum. *Mmm.* Feel the vibration of sound enter your chest and penetrate your heart with its loving touch. If you like, you may add a vowel with the *mmm*, following whatever sound feels satisfying: *ahmmm, eeemmm, uuummm,* or *ooommm. OM,* of course, is the best-known mantra (from Sanskrit) used for meditation in the Hindu traditions. They say this is the sound emitted by the universe, a song that unites all forms within creation. You can tweak it slightly to *home* and feel your heart merging with its home in the cosmos.

When you come to silence, dwell in the residual internal vibrations, the resonance within your heart. Taking time to bathe in the aftereffect of the sound is just as important as the sounding itself. Alternate several times between the sound and the silence.

&? GOING FURTHER

Bathe in Light

Meditators sometimes spontaneously have a sense of being flooded with light, as though a waterfall of light flows down all around and inside of them. This experience can also be invited and cultivated.

You can do this sitting or lying down, either indoors or outdoors. Begin by remembering a time when you were bathed in light and loved the feeling—at the seashore, at a river or lake, on a mountain, possibly at sunrise, late morning, or early afternoon. The light could have been the delicate radiance from the moon and stars. What you want to find is the sense of being delighted, as if the cells of your body know and cherish the light. Taking a minute or more to recall this enjoyment will remind you of what a natural pleasure light can be. Everyone has a different way of approaching these experiences. When you savor these favorite memories, the nuances of your own sensory pathways are highlighted.

What is the quality of light that you love? What sensations do you feel on your skin? What do you feel in your eyes? How does it feel to breathe when bathed in sunlight? How deeply into your body do you want the light to penetrate?

Now bring your attention to the space above you and notice what's there. If you are sitting, explore the sensations at the top of your head. If lying on your back, sense the area all above the front of your body and face. Imagine that a source of light hovers somewhere above you in a way that you thoroughly enjoy. Let it be as close or as far, as radiant or gentle, as natural or supernatural, as you like. Imbue it with any color you crave.

Bathe in this quality of light; let the light wash through you and around you. Let your senses open to it; feel your particular relationship to this quality as it nourishes, cleanses, and illuminates. Invite the light in and receive its gift. Through this communion, know your luminous being.

Your Secret Prayer

Create or select a favorite prayer and learn it by heart. Get comfortable in the energy of the prayer. No one will hear you, so let it be as mushy or as powerful as you dare.

To prepare yourself, light a candle if you like, or create an altar or a special arrangement of the room. You may want to use images of space, nature, or a goddess such as Kwan Yin, Mother Mary, or Kali.

Sit comfortably and establish your inner sanctuary (as described earlier). When you are ready to meditate, gently bring the prayer into your mind. Speak the words out loud, sing them, or voice them internally. Say the prayer over and over, letting the meaning penetrate through your soul. Then sit in the silence and continue to feel.

At any time you may get the impulse to move, so of course let that happen. You may sway or dance with the words, or your hands may come together in the prayer mudra, or they may take on other meaningful gestures. Your spirit is moving you.

❧ REFLECTIONS

- Notice the effect of giving yourself sanctuary. Is there more relaxation in your body, a little more space? You may experience an emotional relief, gratitude, glee, or defiant satisfaction.

- Did you find a residual tendency to apologize for taking time and space, or a furtive guilt? If so, don't feel guilty about that! Just ask, "What old rules am I breaking? Which can I now release?"

- Remember a time when you were in a scary situation and you dealt with it somehow; then, when you got home and were safe, you had the shakes and let yourself fall apart. You realized all the bad things that could have happened, and you trembled and cried. Instinctively, this is the way it's supposed to be: in an emergency we function well, then later we let go of the stress. Taking the time to heal is important; otherwise our emergency resources become depleted. Honor this healing instinct.

- You can let a mantra or prayer continue silently inside you throughout the day. During times of great transition, this is a powerful way to underscore the new vibration you are moving into.

❧ SECRET #6
ANSWER THE CALL

What do I need today?
I need to stretch before I meditate, that much I know.
Organic movement, not specific—something from within.
The last thing I want right now is to be controlled.
Okay, I'll do the "slinky thing" stretch, with some easy rhythmic music.

Lie on the ground, give over my weight, begin to reach and roll . . .
Feel my whole body awakening, muscles unwinding in pleasure,
Slowly, gently finding the flow.
Oh sigh and groan, oh joyous moan—ooph, this feels so good.
I curl and spread, unfold like some strange exotic life form
Opening into the jungle heat.

Yes, the call of the wild . . . Rrrrr . . .
Let me loose, set me free, give me space to breathe!
I wrestle out of my false constraints—my arms draw close, then stretch far,
Legs pull in, press out again with primitive power.
My breath is fierce . . . panting like an animal, pulsing like a flame.
I'm a force of nature—savage, raw, untamed!

Whew . . . I'll slow down now, pause to feel the dance within.
The air crackles with electricity. . . . My body is on fire.
Every finger streams with life force, every toe and hair . . .
My belly and heart stir with desire . . .
Desire for freedom, and . . . uh-oh, I admit it—power.
Ha! That's a taboo breaker, right there. Om- . . . ni- . . . po- . . . tence!

Now what does that mean? What's the true desire?
The freedom of full expression and the power to expand,
For you to see me—all of me—and celebrate me as I am.
Oh, I get it. It's up to me first: I can celebrate me. I can expand in love . . .
I don't want to be controlled, nor can I control how you think about me.
But I can endorse myself. I can let my energy flow . . .
That is the power. That is the freedom. Let me breathe with that. . . .

The flame of passion pulses in my core, this I know.
I am full now, and free—full with the power of life.

🙾 🙾 🙾

REJOICE IN DESIRE

The body and psyche want our wholeness and continually offer us healing messages. Listening to their wisdom is a skill and an art.

When we have desires or cravings, life is calling us toward what will
replenish and recharge us. All living things turn toward their sources of
energy and nourishment, like a plant turning toward the sun and
extending its roots down toward water. Meditation is a "tropism," an
instinctive turning toward nutrients for our soul. Approached in this
way, meditation is juicy and dynamic.

People usually think of meditation as a mental discipline, with a
dry, clinical tone. Meditating in this dissociative mind-set can lead to a
peaceful but slightly depressed and devitalized existence. Your desires
are your compass; they point you in the direction you need to go. The
word *desire* means "from a star." You are following your star. This is why
people who cut themselves off from desire become disoriented—a danger all the more likely to befall those who meditate in a "spiritual" tone.
Inside every desire is a longing for spiritual experience. That is why
meditation is not about detachment but rather about entering our
desires, letting them lead in toward the self as well as out toward the
world.

A healthy approach to meditation is one in which you answer an
inner call. Sometimes an inner part of you is calling for attention.
Sometimes your Self is calling you. The part of you that is reading this

book is on a quest. Be with your questions. Inhabit your inquiry. You will be led through to the answer, fulfilled not just in words and thoughts but in the rearrangement of your being.

A Cauldron of Fire

When we make time for ourselves in meditation, we get in touch with the deepest callings of the heart—the "heart's desire," the aching joy of something yet to be manifested. The aching is hard to take, but that is what meditation is really for, to give us the serenity to live with a full heart.

Consider that human passion is a reflection of divine passion, the force that propels consciousness to unfold. Your desires and passion guide you to the heart of your life. They put you in conversation with the universe. Within desire is psychic and physical energy, and passion is what makes meditation lively and meaningful. You are collaborating with creation to be able to give what is yours to give, and to receive.

The heart is not just sweetness and light, violins and valentines. It is a heated cauldron, an alchemical vessel of transformation. Within its fiery walls the opposites meet and mate. It is a dance of passion between life and death, love and hate, sorrow and joy, pride and shame, hope and despair. It takes courage to admit what is in your heart; there is so much to feel. But this mating, with all its intensity, gives birth to your visions and dreams. Accept the challenge and let yourself be transformed. Dance with the fires of creation and breathe with the intensity. Step into the pyre willingly, cackle and roar with the flames.

Passionate women (and who isn't one, really?) are similar in some ways. They care deeply. They are curious. They are willing to love, to be moved, to engage with life, and to suffer its realities. They are sojourners in the mysterious adventure of being human, open and courageous despite their fear.

When Jennifer (whom you met in the first chapter) first began private sessions, she said that she felt numb, even though she knew there were lots of feelings just under the surface. She had participated in some "Moving Theater" workshops with me, and a few months later she decided to explore some more. Despite weekly talking therapy, her energy felt blocked. Jennifer is a thirty-five-year-old single mother with a five-year-old son and has a new and challenging job in computer technology sales. Blond and classically pretty, she described a pattern of getting involved with men who could not commit to relationship. We began by just sitting and having her pay attention to her inner sensations. After a while she reported a sense of fullness, as if she were about to explode. I suggested that she move with this feeling, so she jumped up and started to dance, making large sweeping gestures with her arms and stalking around the room. Her exhalations turned into catlike sounds that seemed to clear out the space around her, making more space for her to breathe.

As energy moved through her body, she realized that she felt shame for taking up so much space, for her anger, and for her desires. I asked her to pause and sense the currents of life flowing through her. She stretched her arms wide and breathed, quivering with emotion. I said very softly, "You have so much love in you, Jennifer, so much passion." With that, the floodgate opened, and tears streamed down her face. "Yes!" she exclaimed, "I feel so strongly, I have so much love to give. I adore my son. I am excited about my career. I want to make a difference in the lives of people I know. I want someday to share my love with a man, but the important thing is, I can feel the passion of my own heart, now, in my own life!" Embracing her passion became Jennifer's ongoing meditation—to take fifteen minutes in the morning to sit or stand and breathe with the fullness. What had felt like numbness was actually an intensity that was difficult to accept. It is not always easy to tolerate the power of our love.

Get intimate with the nuances of your passion. What do you love? What do you suffer? The experience is extremely personal, and it helps to recognize that your version may be very different from someone else's. Passion can be wild, outward, and vocal or subtle, inward, and refined—or a mixture of both. For some women their passion is not about specific issues or activities but resides in an inner connectedness that is like a quiet and steady flame. For others it is a blazing fire—zeal for a cause, all-consuming ambition, or the zest to live at full throttle with no holds barred. Some women know their passion best through personal intimacy or commitment to family; others channel it in enthusiasm for the arts, whether as patrons or as artists.

Let meditation be a bonfire of the heart to endorse the very particular way that passion is expressed through you. Shakti, Aphrodite, Artemis, Kali, Kwan Yin—whom does your passion serve?

Cravings

Everyone has cravings. These hungers are a primary way our instincts tell us what we need. When you tune in, you'll undoubtedly notice a craving for something: rest, nourishment, love, play, excitement, silence, solitude, companionship, touch, some kind of treat.

When you relax in meditation, what you crave will be right in your face. So face it. No matter what shows up, don't push it away. You are not a bad person for having the craving; you are not weak or infantile. Your instinct for self-balancing is asserting itself. Get curious; learn from the desire. Let the yearning take you right into the heart.

If a craving has gone long unfulfilled—if we were not permitted to satisfy it in childhood, for example—it can bring up pain when finally met. We have learned to turn away from the desire, so we don't trust it. We put a crusty shell around such a desire. The body turns against it, encapsulates it. The desire itself can even seem like an enemy. We've adapted—who needs it? But deep inside the lack is like an injury, a limp, or a broken wing that cannot heal. We are out of balance. When we don't know how to meet the real craving, we often replace it with something else that doesn't quite work and may even be harmful. This is the root of addiction. When we really need rest, we work harder or turn to alcohol or drugs; when we really need love, we overeat; when we really need touch, we get addicted to sex; when we feel deprived, we buy more stuff. Our personalities are built around our unfulfilled needs and cravings.

❧ VONDA'S SWEETNESS

Vonda is a beautiful storyteller, versed in the ancient female ways. She is a big woman with a big aura and big feelings. Over the years she has found ways to keep her energy moving, though managing her intensity remains a great challenge. Despite her desperate desire to lose weight, the more she has struggled with it, the more she has gained. This, of course, has caused her to suffer tremendously.

Recently in class we all danced with what we crave. We had opened ourselves up in movement and then slowed down to tune in. Slowly each woman began to let her inner desire unfold. At one point I glanced over at Vonda and noticed her tears. But soon she was dancing with a radiant smile and making playful eye contact with others as her movement flowed. After class she exclaimed, "Today I finally realized what I've been craving all along—my own sweetness. I can feel it now. Camille, this is so big!"

Staying in touch with her sweetness has become one of Vonda's ongoing meditations. Vonda was astonished that a state so natural could seem so radical, and felt she was breaking a powerful taboo. She is not alone; for women to dwell in their essential being is a revolutionary and deeply creative act.

Admitting what we deeply crave stretches and challenges who we think we are. We may even feel ashamed. The personality can adapt heroically to unfulfilled desire, but then identifies with a false strength. To become more whole is a death to the old self, and it can be terrifying. But the relief from that heroic stance, the melting of the shield around the heart, and the gratification of its longing, bring a rich contentment that is more than worth the struggle.

LONGING FOR THE DIVINE

There are desires and longings that seem overtly spiritual—longing for the sacred, the divine, the eternal, the infinite. These emerge from a profound hunger in the soul, a craving so great it cannot be fulfilled by anything in ordinary life, and yet it cries to be addressed. Many people in recovery have said that their drug or alcohol addiction was based in an unacknowledged longing for spiritual experience. In meditation, if you let it, your longing for the divine spreads your heart wide open.

The craving may be for intimate connection with the inner Beloved. The yearning for mystical union, or alchemical *conjunctio,* is an archetypal desire—structured into the psyche itself. It may seek fulfillment with a human partner, or in inner marriage with the Divine Self, Krishna, or Christ.

In 1982, I was immersed in sacred solitude, a time of marrying my Self. In the depths of those winter nights in Santa Fe, I would put on my ceremonial black dress and muse in front of the fireplace sipping sake, burning for union with God. I'd dance in a wild passion, wailing and roaring at my failures in human relationship and devoting myself to love divine. Slowly my heart was rendered, torn open with grief, and made ready to be penetrated. The inner lover became an ecstatic reality, not just spiritual but deeply erotic. I no longer looked to an external source; I was complete within myself. I'd walk the moon-kissed snowy streets and sing to the Beloved, pacing my steps to the rhythm of my simple song. I'd meditate long hours with its chant flowing through me like a mantra. Devotion is a powerful magnet, and surprising in its results. Lorin came into my life that full moon in January 1983. Coincidence or magic—who's to say? With him, then, I was able to share from this wholeness. Of course, such full engagement brought its own fiery challenges, but we'll save those tales for another time!

It has been said that a woman's nature is devotional. This is true for many women, or true at certain times of their lives. They devote themselves wholeheartedly to their children, to their mate, to their friends, to God, or to spiritual teachers as proxies for God. Dedication to a cause, to your creativity, or to your career is also a kind of devotion. Meditate with the passion of your devotion as it kindles the depth of meaning and connection you crave. Let its flame warm and nourish your entire being, then radiate that warmth out into the world.

WHEN SHE CALLS

There are times in our lives when we need to see the feminine face of God. Though the divine is beyond definition, exclusively male concepts of the godhead are alienating for women. A female sense of divinity makes it much easier for us to identify the sacred within ourselves—an essential aspect of our spiritual health. Many women have found healing, solace, inspiration, and empowerment in opening to the Goddess.

When we open to the *state of being* we call the Goddess, we experience the sacred all around us in every form of life. All of creation is Her body, and we are embraced within it. To enter into communion with Her is to be in a state of grace, inside the Body of Love. Held by Her, the processes of birth and death are understood as part of the eternal, transformative cycle of creation. Emotions, from ecstasy to grief, are Her dance, the forever-unfolding, self-resurrecting movement of love.

It is reassuring to find that in cultures all over the world and throughout the ages, female images of deity abound. In ancient times, when humans were in closer rapport with nature, and perhaps more obviously dependent on it, the image of God was feminine. Female icons and statues of goddesses have been found at archaeological sites dating back to 25,000 B.C. In simpler, earthier times, the sense of the sacred was immanent and immediate, not disembodied, transcendent, and something to be found "elsewhere." Indigenous cultures still carry this wisdom. In the later history of Western culture, female divinity was literally buried, but there is now a resurgence of this knowledge.

The classical goddesses and other female archetypes represent different aspects of the feminine, and they are powerful teachers. Each of these sacred images embodies a message, a feminine truth, a certain vibratory reality. If you long to embody a particular energy, meditating on the goddess of that aspect will open you to the quality she carries. Sometimes, especially in times of transformation, a goddess may call you! When a new perspective or sense of meaning is required, a goddess (quality or energy) may *insist* that you hear her wisdom.

In this section we name some of the female images of deity that women meditators most often refer to and have found meaningful. (There are many in-depth descriptions in other sources. See the references at the back of the book.) As you read about their attributes, see if any of them call to you:

- Kwan Yin (Chinese) or Tara (Tibetan)—mercy, compassion, healing
- Shakti (Indian)—creativity, life force, "to be able to"
- Kali (Indian)—goddess of fire, fierce protection, the death of illusion
- Sophia (ancient Greek)—wisdom, inner knowing
- Aphrodite (ancient Greek)—beauty, sensuality, erotic love
- Artemis (ancient Greek) and Diana (Roman)—independence, adventure, living in the wild
- Hecate (ancient Greek)—solitude, truth, cutting away the false
- Lilith (Hebrew)—autonomy, defiance (Adam's first mate)
- Shekinah (Hebrew)—She who dwells within; immanence
- Changing Woman (Navajo)—She who walks in beauty; transformation

THE CALL OF THE WILD

There is an untamed part of you, not owned by anyone. Inside you are mountains, streams, volcanoes, thunderstorms, broad vistas, and meadows filled with flowers. There are birds there, and bears, wildcats, buffalo, and deer. This is your inner nature's wildlife preserve. Stay close to it, because connection to this wildness is absolutely essential. If you feel used up or overworked, if you have given too much or been too much in control, your inner wildness may call to you—loudly!

You are a force of nature—accept it. Deny your wildness at your peril—it is an essential key to your vitality. Meditation is not to tame you but to set you free! Learn from the Greek goddess Artemis—archetype of the huntress—attuned to nature, unfettered and strong. Reclaim your freedom and power. Rejoice in the primal energy of joyous excitement, sexuality, aggression, and passion. Make room for these fiery qualities in your meditation. Dance to primitive drum music and then meditate. Conjure up your wild spirit and breathe with it during meditation. Hear and answer the Call of the Wild.

❧ EXPLORATIONS

- List cravings you occasionally have. What are the similarities among them?

- If you could magically transport yourself to some wilderness environment, where would you go? What qualities would it provide? (for example, nurturance, adventure, freedom, solitude, inspiration)

- What natural environment matches your sense of being wild and free? (for example, crashing waves, a waterfall, the wind dancing in the trees, a high mountain peak, a volcano)

- In what activities are you most liberated? When have you been most untamed? Take the memory of these times into your meditation.

- How do you experience passion? When have you been impassioned? When you're in love? Angry? Sexual? Inspired? What do you feel strongly about? What are the nuances of your passion, the internal texture, qualities of movement, the particular feeling tones?

- The dark passions are so painful that we want to turn away, detach from them or wash them out, but they provide important clues to our true longing. Envy, jealousy, and wrath are signals from some area in your life that needs attention. When have you felt envy? What quality do you see in that person that you want to develop in yourself? In what way can you move toward the state of being they represent? How can you recognize your own version of that quality? Perhaps the message is to value yourself, the choices you've made, and the life you have created.

- What is a desire you wholeheartedly embraced that turned out well? Perhaps you traveled far to see a friend or family member and the richness of that meeting still warms your heart. Perhaps you took a risk in starting your own business, or creating a work of art.

- When have you gone after one desire and attained it, only to realize that you wanted something else?

- Have you ever successfully killed a desire?

- Make a list in your journal of fifty desires that would be fun to fulfill—both realistic and fanciful desires. Be extravagant, excessive, and imaginative: *I want a new lacy nightgown. I want that blue silk dress. I want dinner at the most expensive restaurant in town. I want a thick new Persian carpet. I want a promotion. I want my own company. I want to own my house free and clear. I want a secret cabin on the side of a mountain where I can go to be alone. I want the perfect mate. I want a month in Tahiti. I want to win the Oscar, the Grammy, the Nobel Prize. I want suitcases full of hundred-dollar bills. I want to be president . . .*

SKILL CIRCLE #6: HOW TO MEDITATE WITH DESIRE

Inside every desire is a movement toward something, a *reaching outward* to grasp what you want or to expel what you do not want. It is also a *movement inward*, to take in and hold close what you desire. In meditation we can appreciate the movement of desire while remaining in a luxurious state of rest. This combination of restfulness and electricity is healthful and to be cultivated. Knowledge of your desire—no matter how intense, unrealistic, fantastic, unattainable, or politically incorrect—gives you important information; it can even be more fun to explore the craving than to have the craving fulfilled. When you meditate, give yourself permission to dive into that intensity. Enter it fully so that it can teach you how to be fulfilled.

If you think of a quality for even one minute a day in meditation, you build that into your awareness: balance, serenity, inner strength, love, delight, zest, sexual magnetism, or even focus itself—whatever quality you feel you need, crave, or want to play with. When you put your attention on the word standing for the quality you seek to embody,

WARM-UP: A MANDALA OF DESIRES

Make a chart or painting of your primary desires: love, peace, cosmic connection, power, fortune, relationship, freedom. Find images in magazines, paint, draw, or simply write them in some way. Arrange them within a circle, like slices of a pie. This is a visual display of how all the desires coexist and reflect your whole self. A mandala is a representation of the psyche; the self resides at the center, surrounded by other levels of being. In Tibetan Buddhism, for example, those parts are imagined as wrathful or benevolent deities. The initiate meditates on those images to incorporate their energies. Do the same with your desires.

you alert your body and nervous system to learn about and surprise you with that quality. It will start showing up in your life spontaneously. The process of focusing on the quality of desire is instinctive: bathing in the feeling, singing it, feeding on it, or being massaged by it.

Getting Inside a Desire

- What do you crave? What is the image of the desire?
- What quality of energy does it provide?
- How would you experience yourself if the desire were satisfied? How would your body feel? How would you breathe? Take some time to ponder this.
- What is the tone of the energy—dense or gossamer, dark or light? Do you see any colors? Is its movement fast or slow, direct or indirect? Does the energy move up, down, forward, back, out, or in? Is it fiery, passionate? Or does it simmer warmly inside you like a quiet flame? Is it an ache, a soulful, soft longing? Is the tone soothing, nourishing? Or is the force angry, explosive, purgative?
- Allow the impressions of the energy to permeate you. Let every cell and fiber drink in those qualities. Cherish these new sensations.

Dance the Movement of Desire

You can do this as a meditation in itself, or before or after meditating. Sitting, standing, or lying down, start with your hands on your chest or belly. Acknowledge the desire, all of those impressions. When you're ready, slowly unfold, letting your arms extend outward, in whatever direction your desire takes you. Reach way out for what you want, or push away what you don't. Then draw back in, gathering what you do want into yourself. Let your hands touch your belly, heart, or anywhere else that is craving. Pause for a moment to let your body receive the quality you crave; really take it in. To "give body" to your desire through movement is to experience even more of its intensity. If emotion comes, accept it. Laugh, cry, growl, sing, or roar if you want to. Continue alternately reaching out and gathering in. You can breathe with the movement, exhaling with the outward flow and inhaling as you draw in. To inhale is to receive life, and you can imbue the breath itself with the particular tone you crave. Don't worry about coordinating the movement and breath if that is too complicated.

The desire may take you traveling through the room, so let your feet be free to move too. Experiment with different tempos of movement, faster or slower. Then gradually come to a pause in either position (reaching or gathering), a sculptural pose that captures the intensity. Breathe in that shape, with all that it evokes. Sense the movement of energy that continues within this apparent stillness. Then, when you are satisfied, gently release. Take one more deep inhalation, then exhale into a relaxed position, standing, sitting, or lying down. You can go on into further meditation, or make a gentle transition into your next activity. Take a few minutes to imagine moving through your world informed by this desire.

ᕕ MEDITATIONS

Longing for the Divine

Breath is inspiration. With every inhalation you take, you are permeated with Spirit, pneuma, prana, life itself. When you bring awareness to this ongoing movement, you are literally inspired. Even one conscious breath can infuse your whole being with the quality of the sacred that you crave. Dwelling in this receptive state for a full meditation is truly divine.

Find a position that allows you to be open and relaxed. Feel free to invent new postures. Let your eyes open or close, as you feel called. When you've settled in, begin to invoke the aspect of the divine that you long for. Is it unconditional love, a sense of the eternal, solace for your tired soul? Is it creative inspiration, mystical union, or cosmic consciousness? Explore the particular feeling. Do you have an image of deity—the Beloved, the universe, Christ, Nature, the Great Mother, a goddess or god? Is there something you long to hear, or something you want to express—perhaps a prayer? Be surprised by your response.

As you pay attention to the quality of contact you desire, its energy will begin to suffuse you. Know that the divine, by definition, is always present with you—as intimate and immediate as your breath. It is the giver of life. Imagine how that Sacred Presence surrounds you and saturates the entire space, the air, the ground.

Consecrate each breath to that awareness. As you inhale, imbue the breath with divine essence; receive it into your body and heart. As you exhale, let your own essence flow out to rejoin that source. Continue with the conscious flow in and out, a deepening loop of connection. Feel how with each inhalation and exhalation divine breath enters you, gathers you up into itself, and weaves you into the tapestry of life.

The Call of the Wild

These exercises can be done sitting, standing, or lying down.

Inner Wilderness Choose a wilderness environment that calls to you, as you identified earlier under "Explorations." What qualities do you crave? Imagine yourself there; become immersed in the internal imagery. Let your inner senses open up as you take in the sounds, sights, smells, and textures of the image.

What is the quality of light? Sunny, shaded, dappled, or dark like the night sky? What colors do you see in this environment? What sounds do you hear—the wind, the sound of water, birds or insects? What is the texture of the air—cool and breezy, hot and dry, warm and sultry? How does it smell—resinous, flowery, rich like soil? Is the space expansive and mostly open, dense like a forest, or containing and nestling like a cave? In the image, do you want to stand, run, fly, lie down, kneel, or sit? What are the sensations of that inner action? How do you breathe? What pleasures do you sense as you imagine yourself there?

Drink in all of these impressions; receive the nourishment, calmness, or power. Let your whole body feel the mini-vacation of this time away in your inner wilderness.

Wild and Free Choose the natural phenomenon that matches your feeling of being wild and free or creates the quality of energy that you crave. Meditate on becoming that force of nature. Perhaps it is the wild freedom of a rushing river or a cleansing wind, the expansive heat of a roaring flame, or the explosive energy of a volcano.

Acknowledge the power and dynamism of this natural phenomenon. What are the particular qualities of its energy and movement?

What internal texture does its movement create? Does it make a sound? As you see, hear, or feel the image, merge with those impressions.

Give over completely to the inner qualities, whatever they are. Let the vital energy of your image come right into your body. You may be sitting still, but inside you is the rush or gush or swirl of unconfined natural power. (If you get the urge to dance its wild energy, see "Dance Your Passion" under "Going Further.") Open to the sensations of natural life force as it streams through you, and let it cleanse and revitalize every cell.

🕃 GOING FURTHER

Welcome All Desires

This is a good technique to do in a group, if you have the courage to admit what your desires really are and to speak freely.

Under "Explorations" you made an extravagant list of desires. Now sit somewhere with the list in a meditative way. One by one, pick a word or phrase from each desire and speak it to yourself. As you say the word, notice what you feel in your body—your belly, your heart, and your skin. You may be surprised at how intense it is to embrace your desires. The idea is to welcome all of your desires completely, no matter how unrealistic or forbidden. Cherish them, and let them melt right into your body.

Continue for about five minutes. Then pause and let yourself be carried away. What tends to happen is that the mind spontaneously falls into quietness as a rest from the intensity. Some days you may find yourself afraid to articulate your desires or to feel grief because they remain unfulfilled. You may feel tremendously excited by desire and interpret that excitement as restlessness and an inability to meditate.

This exercise does three things:

1. It lets meditation be a home for your desires and for anything new that wants to develop in you.

2. It trains you to sense the sensations and energies underneath the desire. Often we experience only the image or end result of desire, but its energies are more fluid and can be shaped.

3. It links your inner and outer worlds.

Heart's Desire Meditation

To be able to tolerate your heart's desire requires courage, safety, compassion, and perseverance—basically, all the resources you have. How close are you to your heart's desire? What do you ache for? When you are ready to hear its call, enter the fire of the heart.

As directed in the skill circle, you can get inside your desire. When you let yourself feel the yearning, what do you notice? Bring your attention to your chest and enter your heart. What are its sensations? Is there an image or picture of your heart's desire? Notice the sensory detail. How does the energy of the image move? How would you feel if it were fulfilled?

Meditate with the image and sensations of energy. Dance the movement. Let the longing stretch your heart open and teach you how to live to your fullest expression.

Dance Your Passion You can track your passion specifically with the suggestions in the skill circle for dancing with desire. But sometimes a general craving in your body to dance freely has no particular content at first but becomes more specific as you move. Either way, give your passion carte blanche to be expressed.

Put on some music that matches your inner mood and begin to breathe with the rhythm and feeling it evokes. Let the urge to dance take over your whole body. Begin to move the part of your body that feels it the most: your hands, your feet, your hips, your spine. Maybe it's your mouth that wants to let out some primal breath or sound. Let the energy build. How free can you be? Get wild: stomp the ground, shake your booty, make large dramatic gestures with your arms. Give over to the ache of longing as you reach out and draw in. Surrender to your passion!

After ten minutes or so gradually slow down to a pause and bring your awareness inside. Keep breathing consciously as you come to apparent stillness. Savor the ecstatic sensations as energy circulates all through your body.

❧ REFLECTIONS

- What do you find especially satisfying as you welcome your desires?
- As you did the "Explorations," were you surprised by your response?
- What new insights do you have about yourself?
- In what way can you cultivate your heart's desires?

❧ SECRET #7
RIDE YOUR RHYTHMS

I know this feeling.

Breasts full and ponderous,

Belly bulging, about to burst.

Any minute now, blood will ooze between my thighs.

Just don't poke me, I might sprout a leak.

Heavy, sloggy, huge . . .

Like I've just crawled out of some deep dark lagoon.

That's it! My earliest ancestor: the primeval pond of creation.

Glug, glug, glug . . . oh, yeah.

The unlikely origin of life, rising up out of the goo—

Gurgles and spurts of cells becoming bodies, bodies becoming mates . . .

Eons of little deaths and births, all the chance meetings

That created us here, in this moment, now.

Surge, gush, surge, gush . . . the flow through every female—

My mother, her mother before her, all the way back—

An unbroken chain of blood

Since the very beginning of time . . .

Change, change . . . Woman, thy name is change.

Man, what we go through!

Oh, heavy body, you carry this history inside you—

Heaving through this heart,

Sloshing around in this pelvic bowl.

I won't resist . . . I give in to the weight.

I sit on the Earth, as the Earth—clay upon clay.

Ah, I see . . . I am a vessel, a vehicle of the mystery:

Blood flows, life flows, time flows through . . .
The ancient transformative rhythms this body knows.

And as I remember this sacred secret now
My womb begins to smile . . .

❧ ❧ ❧

FEMININE MYSTERIES

Our bodies know about change, rhythm, and cycles. This is women's eternal, universal secret. Nature is rhythm, and our bodies are part of nature—not only the immediate earth environment but the exquisite vast movement of the cosmos. Cosmic connection and interdependence for us are not abstract ideas; they are in our bodies, up close and personal. Through our blood rhythms and responsiveness to the seasons and the moon, women live right inside the transformative cycles of life.

Female biology puts us in touch with life's deepest rhythms—the dance of birth, death, and renewal. Through the metamorphoses of menstruation, motherhood, and menopause, women directly experience the cyclical fecundity of nature. Men do not share this body knowing; these are women's mysteries. Each phase of a woman's life—youth, fertility, midlife, elderhood—has its special gift and is an initiation into some aspect of the mystery. Mothers, for example, often speak of pregnancy and birth as a spiritual transformation, a surrender in body and soul to the flow of creation and their place within it. There is an undeniable rapport between mother and child. In breast-feeding, nipples gush with milk in silent synchronization with the baby's hunger—even when the mother is a hundred miles away. For women, intuition and communion are not abstract goals or ideals but accessible, indisputable, and commonly experienced facts of life.

The morphing of a woman's body within these cycles of fertility is a kind of shape-shifting. Think of it: each month, for decades, we swell and bleed from our wombs. In pregnancy we are dramatically altered as our bodies and psyches give over to the needs of the strange, magical creature inhabiting us. In menopause we decompose and recompose into some new form entirely—at least that's how it feels. Women shape-change. It's a matter of course, the course of matter. No wonder women have been called witches and inspired fear. How can men possibly understand what a woman's body goes through? They have no idea!

Georgianne Cowan, a mother and artist, writes of pregnancy in her essay "The Sacred Womb":

The impetuous seed of creation does not exactly come forth on little cat feet. Rather, it takes hold without deliberation. A woman's womb, once virginal except for the cleansing rivers of menstrual blood flowing through her, becomes possessed by this amazing force of life. A new sensation flutters inside, a veritable stranger takes up residence inside its mother's belly. The queen has allowed one of two million insistent sperm into her domain, and there is no turning back as cells divide and the royal egg transforms from zygote to blastocyst. The force of life is aggressive and steadfast as the embryo recapitulates the stages of evolution. The throes of this alchemy unfurl a sensitive sea-like creature who develops a tail, fins, and eventually tendrils of arms and legs. For 266 days inside the womb, the mysteries of the life-cycle are enacted as the initial protoplasm expands, forms, and blossoms.

Who is this new visitor? What is this oscillating, fluid mystery inhabiting her body? Is it human or vegetable, monster or something completely unknown to our collective psyches? The *stranger* takes on a somewhat ominous quality, simply by the nature of its invisibility. Who is to know what is forming inside? The answer may rest in our collective knowing, on the faith that our species gives birth to its own and will eventually birth a human being. Is it not unlike our faith in the return of spring after a winter of darkness? In the velvet womb of the earth, in the dark womb of our soul, we've peered into the shadowed void of the unknown and trusted that from fallow fields of dormancy will spring new life.

Women's bodies and psyches are deeply attuned to the waxing and waning cycles of nature, the phases of the moon, and the seasons. The lunar pull on oceans and tides moves within us, in the inner tides of emotion and body fluids. That the word *menses* is related to *moon* and *month* is no big surprise. The four terrestrial seasons of growth, harvest, decomposition, and rebirth reflect an internal psychic rhythm as well. Growth is a process with its own inexorable timing, an ebb and flow that cannot be forced but can be tended and trusted to unfold. Women know this from the inside out. The cycles of life are relentless and powerful. When human beings try to control them, we suffer; when we cooperate, we thrive. Such is nature's design, so we may as well acquiesce. These natural cycles are all interconnected and affect us whether we acknowledge the connections or not. Their rhythms literally inform us, and it is feminine wisdom to collaborate with them. We must let go. But within that surrender is the key to our strength.

Women are very adaptable; we have brilliantly accommodated to the rigorous pace of modern life and learned how to override our natural rhythms to get the job done. We have an astonishing ability to do a million things at once, and many women are "doing it all." We are out there! This is exhilarating, and I for one love the surge of excitement that comes from dancing at my personal edge. But when the edge becomes a chronic push, it's easy to neglect the inner need and to become depleted and off balance. When our roots spread out too shallow and too far, we lose our ground—the depths of being that are our sustenance and renewal. Let's go for it—no guilt—and let the cup of life be filled. But let's also choose to "say when."

Daily meditation keeps us in touch with these deeper rhythms. Access to the feminine mysteries is as close to us as the womb, as close as our breath, as close as the movement of night and day. If we get the message, we can willingly submit and permit ourselves to be changed. We can surrender to the unraveling that allows a reorganization of our being. If we resist the call, the body and psyche inevitably provide a little boost, getting our attention through sundry physical and psychological symptoms. Hormones are witty messengers. "Female problems" such as PMS are often alleviated when we listen and give in to the call: "Slow down, let go, drop in!" When we do get out of our heads, let go of "doing" and sink down into "being," it is a revelation and a great relief.

In ancient times women's connections to natural cycles were structured with rituals and celebrated. In modern times we can create our own rituals to honor the different cycles going on in our bodies and psyches. In this chapter are explorations to help you attune to these ever-changing needs. You can create meditations that satisfy whatever phase you're in. Within you already are clues to riding these rhythms. Here you will learn how to maximize your natural wisdom.

✥ THE EYE OF THE STORM

Here's some wisdom from a friend of ours, whom we will call Darlene. A chiropractor at the cutting edge of alternative healing, Darlene is a vivacious and sassy redhead who recently passed the sixty-year milestone.

"I meditate when I feel tired, or bad. I go in, and I have the intent to go to the eye of the storm, and I sink into it. One time I was so exhausted I could hardly wiggle. Whatever that itch is, I go into it. Whatever that edge is, I let it tell me what it is. I use the words *softening, melting.* I get completely surrendered, which is like practicing your death. Then when I come back I am remarkably rested, and I feel so much energy has been released. The whole process is tactile; I don't put a story to it. It is a way to practice surrendering.

"One time while traveling in Africa I was so exhausted and cranky that I meditated for three hours, just staying with it, going into the heart of the feeling—surrendering, staying there, melting. I felt like a new person afterward. There is no medication, there is no vitamin, that can bring me back to myself like that."

THE CYCLES OF LIFE

The cycles of life are natural phases that recur within the environment and within us. There are the smaller, quite predictable rhythms of sun and moon—daily, monthly, yearly—and the broader, only somewhat predictable rhythms of the movement of your life from birth to death. There are the eternal cycles of the universe, incomprehensible to our feeble human minds, and there are the minute, frequent, seemingly random, and sometimes equally incomprehensible cycles that every woman undergoes.

Below is a list of the basic cycles of a lifetime. Joan Boryshenko, in her wonderful work *A Woman's Book of Life,* uses the Native American delineation of twelve seven-year cycles. For our purposes, we stick with the four primary rhythms as a simple map. We borrow, however, her salutary term "guardian" for the midlife phase. There is a nifty mythological correlation between the four phases of growth, the seasons, the moon, and certain emotions. Many of us are boomers who will soon be entering the "autumn of our lives," a cliché all the more powerful for its simple truth. Let the clichés of maps such as these stimulate your own creative perception.

- *Youth:* Maiden—spring—birth, new growth, beginnings—crescent moon—anger
- *Fertility:* Mother, artist—summer—full blossom, sexuality, abundance—full moon—joy
- *Midlife:* Guardian—autumn—harvest, ripening, maturity—waning moon—grief
- *Elderhood:* Wise woman, benefactor—winter—decomposition, gestation, letting go—dark of the moon—fear, contraction, retreat
- *Rebirth:* Beginning the cycle again

The seasons provide excellent lessons about our own rhythms and about how each phase nourishes the next. Everybody knows the exuberant rebirth of spring, the fullness and activity of summer, the bittersweet slowing down of fall, the quiet reflection and gestation of winter. There is a psychic reality to these seasonal processes; we require them, and I do not think this is negotiable. People tend to get sick at the change of seasons, a time of enforced retreat when the body must assimilate and adapt. Meditating is a conscious retreat. Here in southern California, where the clues are subtle, I miss nature's dramatic and uncompromising display, so I make the most of every little shift in weather and light. I use the gentlest rain or the barest whiff of cold as full-on winter—an excuse to be cozy, to regenerate, to decompose, to drop down into my roots.

In Oriental medicine different emotions are related to the seasons: anger in spring; joy in summer; grief in fall; fear or retreat in winter. In each season we are prone to imbalances in that emotion, either excess or stagnation. Staying in touch with the flow of emotional and seasonal energy helps to keep us in balance.

The natural rhythms between activity and letting go are innate and instinctive, but how we relate to them is learned behavior. Our mothers and grandmothers were our models, unconsciously affecting our attitudes toward our bodies and their cycles. How we deal with youth, maturity, aging, and death is a product of culture. Angeles Arrien, a Basque teacher and writer on indigenous spirituality, speaks of the four faces of age within us all. Wisdom emerges, she observes, when all four faces are simultaneously present in our awareness. This can be observed in the timeless faces of some people—the child and the crone, the mother and the ingenue—all four in friendly cohabitation within.

The shift from one phase, one face, to another can be challenging. To gaze into the internal mirror with changing eyes is unsettling, to say the least. Energy psychology describes such phase transitions, borrowing a term from physics, as "perturbations." These are the disruptions within a system that precede its potential shift to a higher, simpler order. As human beings, we have the capacity to cooperate consciously with the transformation.

Menopause is a phase transition, notorious for its perturbations. Some women breeze through the menopausal transition; for others it is a tumultuous ride. Its orchestration is as individual as we are. In perimenopause, the usual rhythms of menstruation—and personality—become erratic as the woman's whole being begins the metamorphosis. Hormones, emotions, and self-image enter a wild, creative flux. A woman's identities crack, slough off, and decompose, like outgrown skins, while her new form fights for breath. Fatigue is no stranger; this is a lot of work! She is filled with heat—surges of power that burn away the dross, cleansing and clearing on every level. She may indeed be perturbed—and perturbing—as she grapples with so much change. But from within the apparent chaos, a hidden order eventually emerges—a clarified, simplified state. The crazy dance between the opposites resolves into a third state of integration. Her values reorganize, settling in like a new foundation beneath her feet. With the cessation of monthly periods, her wise blood is retained within herself, transmuted into a new relationship to life. She garners her physical and psychical forces for what she deems important and ruthlessly relinquishes what she does not. She stands tall in her vision, a conscious guardian of life-serving values for her community.

Getting through these perturbations to the new state of freedom and clarity must be the secret in what Margaret Mead called "post-menopausal zest." If we honor the cycle of growth called aging, we "come into our own," as Mark Gerzon describes it in his worthwhile book by that name. Hidden within our language we can find hints of age wisdom. The word *maturity* comes from the Latin for "ripened." We are seasoned with experience, aged like an expensive wine. We are ripe with our sensual knowledge and rich in understanding. These gifts long to be shared. Marta, a writer, designer, and mother of two grown children, is an example of postmenopausal clarity: "My job is to be an observer, to refine my perception and articulate it."

EMILIE'S STORY: "DRAWING FROM A SOURCE BEYOND CULTURE"

At sixty-six, Emilie Conrad, the originator of Continuum movement meditation, is a vibrant, sensuous, and inspiring embodiment of graceful aging. In a recent conversation, Emilie shared: "This is the best time of my life, the full bloom of my existence. Experience and maturation are the bumps and lumps that have helped me to grow. The spiritual source that has fed and sustained me is primary, and without that source, I would not have the strength to learn from adversity.

"I am unmarried at the moment, and love my freedom. My fundamental sensuality is not about someone else, but a lushness within my own organism that is fuller now than when I was younger—richer and more meaningful. In age there is a wrinkled beauty, wisdom, and compassion. The societal onus of aging is huge; a woman feels invisible. The abnegation of a woman's sexuality is disempowering and devastating and it takes tremendous capacity not to be beaten down. Women need to draw from something not culturally based, values beyond what society brings to you. The fortitude is not a physical strength but an existential source. The spiritual connection keeps you ignited. Sexuality and spirituality are so interwoven. Being fed by that well of erotic vitality is a great mystery."

Owning the power of age is tough and shocking. Not owning it only leads to isolation and bitterness. Because youthfulness, especially for women, is such a cultural value, getting older is a particularly rough transition. Women—and their partners—are faced with the challenge of uncharted terrain. There are no maps for this journey.

Far too little is understood and appreciated about the elder phase of life. As a society, we need to hear from older women who have consciously navigated this transition. We are an adolescent culture in many ways, very young in the scheme of the world. As more and more women emancipate themselves in age and share their wisdom and experience, all of us will be enriched.

Here is a composite drawn from the comments and dreams of dozens of women who have made their way through the perturbations:

"I can feel what I am in myself, apart from the needs of others. I have faced the cold and the void. I have made friends with the darkness and the stars. Within the darkness I sometimes feel a wild freedom come over me. I can go outside and dance at night under the stars; I have nothing to fear from the darkness of the woods. I am beyond life and beyond death; I am free. I've seen so much death I no longer fear it; my time will come when it comes. I no longer care what others think of me. I, who had long given up sex and pleasure, discover a new eroticism, a secret intimacy with the stars and the night sky. A mischief and electricity crackles around on my skin. If I could, I would jump on a broom and soar under the stars and laugh. I am free of the need to nurture everybody. The blood that used to flow out in suffering for the world I now hold within myself. I contain my power. I can heal with my herbs or with words of wisdom if I choose, but within myself I am free."

Hecate's Knife

At certain times in a woman's life she must pick up the knife and cut away the cords that bind. There is a feminine instinct to cut, to sever the enmeshments that can imprison a female. It is a balancing instinct, complementary to our relatedness and empathy. All women need periods of solitude to condense into their core. This energy that cuts down to the core is the archetype of Hecate, the Crone, the old and wizened harbinger of the night. Classically the ally of postmenopausal women, Hecate may show up on your path no matter what your age, and she is formidable.

Hecate stands at the crossroads of life, ready to point the way to truth. Her ruthless clarity slashes through the veil of illusion to get to the heart of things. She is the one who frees us from sentimentality, inappropriate relationships, false friends and alliances—and outmoded ways of being. Such unsentimental clarity goes against the myth of feminine sweetness. To discover this dark energy within yourself is startling, but also deeply liberating.

If you are undergoing a radical transformation, Hecate's knife may be just the tool you need. Let her cut away the falseness, let her challenge you to speak the truth arising from your core. Let her teach you the strength of solitude and retreat. There is joy, freedom, and power in aloneness. These resources offer you more choice and freedom in relatedness.

Lorin once remarked: "It is strange that men are so afraid of female freedom. Why? There are a lot of theories, but ultimately it must be that men are not anchored enough in their own power to be able to handle the feminine."

Support the Change

Whatever cycle of transformation you are in, find what supports the change. Transformation is not just a fluffy New Age buzzword; it's a radical challenge to our status quo and fraught with discomfort, especially if we fight it. Can we participate with the urge to change, or will we revert to the supposed security of our familiar self? True change is an act of creation. We pass through the barrier of old taboos into a new state of being. As we cross the threshold, we encounter all our angels and demons. Sometimes it is hard to know which is which. Doubt wrestles with inspiration in a fitful battle of life and death. People around us play their role, often giving voice to our worst fears and self-condemnations. The time of transformation from one state to the next is an extremely vulnerable, delicate transition. Take good care.

Recognize the different state you are achieving, uncomfortable as it may be at first. Endorse the transition; meditate with it. Get used to the new sensations and impressions and resist the temptation to re-create what's "normal." Who's to say? Maybe you will metamorphose into something wondrous, magical, and never before seen, a new creative response to life on earth.

DILATION AND CONTRACTION

The organic rhythm between dilation and contraction is reflected in natural movements everywhere. All the processes of life require the pulsing exchange between these opposite modes. We can look within our own bodies for examples: the dilations and contractions of the uterus and vaginal canal in birthing and orgasm; the open/close throbbing of the heart; the in/out pumping of the breath; the peristalsis of the viscera to excrete and cleanse. Every movement involves the muscular interplay between engaging and releasing. This is true not only physically but also psychologically.

Dilation and contraction reflect the primal rhythm between birth and death. Throughout nature, throughout our bodies, and throughout our psyches, births and deaths are going on all the time. As women, we know this rhythm intimately. We are midwives to birthing and dying; we hold the hands of those who labor to bring life into this world, and the hands of those who are leaving it. We abide with each other through the joys and sorrows of love. We know the paradox that within every birth is the specter of death; within every death is renewal. Each one of us is in the grasp of this movement every moment of our lives, and there is no escape. This is difficult to face. But as we surrender, we are *rendered* in the arms of this reality and brought closer to its breast. This is the heart of the mystery.

Our capacity to go with the movement of dilation and contraction, birthing and dying, shows up internally as an existential sense of fullness or emptiness. You know the half-full or half-empty glass analogy. As with any of the pairs of opposites, the seed of one is in fact within the other. When we do not resist, they continually move and change; emptiness becomes full, and fullness empties, until they are simultaneously one and the same. Dilation becomes contraction, and vice versa; this is the pulse of life. Dilation, the ability to relax, receive, and be filled, spreads us open. Contraction, the ability to engage and express, empties us out. To be fully alive we must find the healthy rhythm between these movements. A hand must release to open before it can clasp what it needs; to gather in, it must muscularly take hold, only to stretch out once again. Can we dilate and be full, receiving from life, from the world? Can we take hold of our lives and shape them? Can we empty out and let go?

Everyone has a personal comfort zone. Some women have grown comfortable staying energetically small; the contracted state feels safe. They are afraid to expand, to take up space and shine in their glory with no apology. Retreat has become habitual, so they lose the traction necessary to follow their desires and birth themselves in the world. Other women fight to be big; they can expand but are afraid to withdraw when they need to, to give in to the little death of letting go. They fill and push, manifesting power and material abundance, but forget how to soften and release. Still others may be trapped in between in a painful paralysis, unable to move in either direction. Each of these styles is an imbalance that creates stress and, ultimately, distress.

Within each breath we die and are born again. When you meditate, you begin to notice your own subtle relationship to that primal rhythm.

Whatever your life is asking of you, it undoubtedly has something to do with dilation and contraction. Ride your rhythms and find the balance, the full movement of both. Stretch a little more into fullness; let go a little more deeply into emptiness. Release the concerns of life, die to the old, and let go. Engage with the passions of life and birth yourself anew in the world. Dare to be empty. Dare to be full.

&% EXPLORATIONS

- When you are emotional, how do you handle yourself? Do you express your emotions? Do you express too little? Too much? Do you feel cleansed afterward?

- What is your general energy level? When you are tired, do you let yourself rest?

- When you have your period, do you allow yourself some time out in the "menstrual hut" to muse and dream? Do you notice that you may be more intuitive when you're bleeding? Take a morning off to feel, to be. You'll find that tension turns into flow.

- Do you experience PMS? If the symptoms could speak, what would they say?

- What phase of life are you in? What does this time seem to ask of you? What are your desires? What are your special needs?

- If you are in perimenopause, how accepting are you about approaching menopause? If you are in menopause, how are you with aging? The cessation of bleeding? The loss of fertility?

- What images and attitudes do you have about getting older? Who has the power?

- Birthing, illness, and death are transformative events. Often we are present for others at these passages; we attend the births, take care of the babies, and administer to the ill and dying. What experiences have you had with birth, severe illness, and death? How have they changed you?

&8 WARM-UP: DANCE YOUR RHYTHMS

Step 1

Identify any of the rhythms going on in your body: fast, slow, lyrical, staccato. Is there a call to rest, to pause in stillness, or to move out with enthusiasm? Do you want to sink down, jump up, run away, draw in, or reach out? Can you feel the beating rhythm of your heart? The natural rhythm of your breath? You can join in this movement. Put a sound track on in your mind, or on the stereo, and let the energy dance. When you give over to the rhythm, notice that it can change from one quality to another.

Step 2

Now bring your attention to the movement of dilation and contraction. Start with one or both hands. Draw your fingers in to make a tight fist, then relax. Stretch them way out, then relax. Play with the rhythm as you continue. Proceed through different parts of your body, tensing the muscles and then releasing, stretching and letting go. Feel how when you tense and then release, the relaxation is even more complete.

Step 3

Feel your whole body as one movement. Extend out through your arms and legs, then curl everything in around your center. Continue alternately reaching out and curling in. If you're using music, let its rhythms slow you down or speed you up. Let your breath speed up or slow down. Every now and then pause in either the extended or contracted position and breathe within it. Then let the pose melt and continue your dance.

When you feel finished or tired, stop the outward movement and relax into a comfortable position—sitting, standing, or lying down. Give over to the dilated state, muscles completely relaxed. Meditate with the relaxation and afterglow of the movement.

&8 SKILL CIRCLE #7:
HOW TO MEDITATE WITH YOUR INNER RHYTHMS

Meditation puts you in touch with the deeper rhythms of your being. It is not about stopping the rhythm.

In every meditation you are plunging into the world of change. Your body goes through a balancing act, rehearsing and reviewing everything you do in a day. The same thing never happens twice. The more you pay attention, the more you perceive this, and the goal is to tolerate all this change. Cultivate a fluid attention that flows with this movement and does not try to control it.

Meditation experience usually changes continuously; nothing stays still. There is a quiet streaming, like the rhythm of breathing, in and out every six or seven seconds. Inside of fifteen seconds you may shift through many thoughts, then feel bodily sensations, then find yourself in silence, then be thinking again. This is often how meditation flows, and your experience is never exactly the same from one moment to the next. You can't step into the same river twice because you are not the same person and it's not the same river. In other words, reality is always fresh and surprising as long as you do not try to impose fixity on your rhythms.

Honor your rhythms. You are different from others in innumerable and important ways. If you violate your natural rhythm, you miss some of the benefits of meditation. Here we offer some suggestions for collaborating with the larger rhythms of life that are always pulsing within. In addition, each meditation will reveal to you the inner rhythms of the moment.

When you sit to meditate, close your eyes and check in with your internal rhythm. Are you slow, a little sluggish, or smooth and flowing? Are you jazzed, frenetic, moving fast like lightning? Investigate your habits. Each person has a range of rhythm. Some people start the day fast and slow down later, some are the opposite. Some are basically fast, some basically slow, some totally steady. The use of addictive substances such as alcohol, tobacco, marijuana, or cocaine is an attempt to find a different rhythm to life. All meditation techniques are about rhythm— of breath, of attention. Breath itself is powerful medicine. Inhalations that are longer than the exhalations are energizing, whereas long exhalations calm.

Some people move fast from fear. Many meditators gain some of the benefits but have never taken on their fear. They hurry in meditation, afraid that they will be punished if they linger. Many teachings suggest that you impose someone else's rhythm on yourself. When you pay attention, you notice many rhythms happening simultaneously, and calling you in different ways as certain rhythmic necessities. While you're sitting there, you may feel the need to make dinner or to get in touch with somebody, or that you need to get in touch with yourself. Your attention moves in a rhythm maybe every four or five seconds, touching one facet of your life and then checking in with another. This is not just your mind wandering. We have to adapt to life, and adapting often is a matter of forsaking our rhythm and learning to move with the herd. If our herd (our school or business) starts at 8:00 A.M., then we have to roll out of bed at 5:00 or 6:00 in order to walk in the door at 8:00. That necessity shapes the rhythm of our day. There are a lot of things you don't have control over. All you can do is get better at organizing yourself and preparing to meet the external demand. People violate their rhythms all the time. If you make meditation another realm where you do this, why bother to meditate?

The Cycles of Waking, Sleeping, and Dreaming

It is truly a necessity to honor the body's rhythm between activity and rest, between stimulation and reflection. Meditation helps keep you rested and ready for action, ready for life, ready for love. This occurs through the alternation of types of rest during meditation. During meditation you cycle through various stages of wakefulness, semi-sleep, deep sleep, and brief snatches of reverie or dreamlike thoughts. If you have a sleep deficit, you probably nod off. (Eventually you pay off the debt.) You know meditation is working when you feel an enhancement in the rhythm of your energy and attention in the flow of your daily life. Your attention is refreshed, and you can ride your rhythms of rest and action with more facility.

Blood Mysteries

Blood rhythms give new meaning to the phrase "go with the flow." Hormones have a kind of crazy wisdom that you can trust. Behind them is internal intelligence; try listening instead of controlling. When hormones are "raging," they exaggerate what's already going on internally as a signal for us to pay attention and learn from it.

Ovulation Many women can sense ovulation. There is often a sharp little pain as the egg moves down the fallopian tube. At midcycle, meditate in celebration of fertility; cherish your womanhood and your creativity. Bask in your juiciness, your ripeness, your sensual power. Let your body open to receive, to be inseminated by life, spirit, love. Let your heart and soul open to your partner in lovemaking, especially if you want to get pregnant. Welcome the new little being into its womb home. And if you do not want to get pregnant, use your discernment and honor your fertility in other ways.

Premenstrual Meditation How do you know you're premenstrual? What are the sensations? If you experience PMS, what are your symptoms? There are many tips for countering the discomfort of PMS (not consuming sugar or caffeine, for example). This information is widely available. But when you do have PMS symptoms, ask them what they want. Whatever the sensations, welcome them in your meditation, strange as that may seem. If you are bloated, give in to the puffy, sloggy feeling. Rather than fight it, be a total blob and give it room to spread. If you are "depressed," let yourself sink down and be vulnerable. Cry for no reason, or watch a sad movie, then meditate. Or if you are irritable, join with the jagged energy. What does it demand? Then negotiate to find a safe and ethical way to satisfy it. Maybe you've been a slave to some outer image, and the symptom is reminding you to come home to yourself. You may need to roar like a lion or dance wildly into a great sweat. Or maybe what you need is space, a little peace and quiet, or simply to sleep!

Menstrual Meditation When your period does come, create some time and space away in your own menstrual hut just to let yourself be. What are the sensations? Are you overheated? Lethargic? Do you have cramps? Whatever the sensations, they require relaxation. Manage to spend as long as you can without having to be on duty, at least the half-hour or so for meditation.

The ancient tribal custom was to sequester menstruating women for days alone or with each other in the "moonlodge." The men may have shunned the bloody mess and feared its primal power, but the women, I'm sure, made the most of the time away. They'd commune with the earth, laugh, drum, and sing. They'd let their blood drip freely into the ground—an offering to their natural origin. When we are bleeding, there is a downward pull to the earth, and the energy actually needs to flow from your pelvis toward your feet. In fact, menstrual discomfort is

🦋 SOME TIPS
FOR RELIEVING
MENSTRUAL
DISCOMFORT

• Take a bath or put
a hot water bottle
on your belly and
relax into the warmth.
Massage your ankles
and heels. (All kinds
of acupressure points
are there for the
female organs—
they're the sore
ones!)

• Try meditating in the
"Double Diamond"
pose. Lie on your
back with your knees
bent out to the side
and the soles of your
feet together in a dia-
mond shape. Bend
your elbows and rest
your hands near your
head. Prop pillows
under your knees or
back for more com-
fort. Meditate in this
double diamond
shape, breathing into
your pelvis, for five to
ten minutes. This
pose releases the
pelvis and allows
excess heat in the
belly organs to dis-
perse. It's also a great
aid to digestion.

usually from congestion of *chi*. Meditate on coming down and in to yourself. Remember Earth as your home and let her hold you. Feel or imagine energy sliding down through your body, away from your head. Let the fullness of your belly and thighs empty through the channels of your legs, swirling through your ankles and out your feet. When you relax into the downward ooze, the sensations often change to a balmy, sensuous connectedness.

Meditation During Perimenopause and Menopause If you are still having periods, all of the PMS and menstrual suggestions remain valuable tools. Research shows that the more positive your attitude toward this transi-tion, the easier your menopausal passage will be. Reframe the changes going on in your body and psyche as an alchemical transformation. Let the fires burn and forge the gold from the lead! Think of hot flashes as power surges, and when one happens, ride the fiery energy. Let it flush out old patterns of holding back and clear new pathways to expressing your truth. You could even let out a riotous yelp or a deep belly bellow of power! Notice how the flashes tend to accompany certain burning thoughts—things you're angry or embarrassed about. They are internal clues to what wants to change.

🦋 TIPS FOR RELIEVING MENOPAUSAL SYMPTOMS

Many of the uncomfortable symptoms associated with dramatic shifts in hor-mone levels can be traced to the liver becoming overtaxed and overheated in pro-cessing them. Let your liver (living!) energy flow. Meditate (either lying down or sit-ting) and focus on your right side beneath the ribs. Give that area more space with your breath, or by stretching slightly to lift and open. Imagine or feel that the liver is relaxing and spreading, sending its heated gift of energy down to your right big toe and up to the top of your head. Say yes to the power streaming all through your right side, and let it expand outward from your body, becoming huge. Then let your left side receive it as well, circulating all the way down to your left big toe.

On the other hand (or foot), you may crave soothing, cooling, and calming. If so, do meditations that remind you of your core strength and serenity—simplicity or sanctuary meditations that disengage you from external demands. Choose whatever mode suits the rhythm you're in, whatever feels right for the moment, and find the pleasure therein.

Moon Mysteries

Lunar consciousness is traditionally the realm of the feminine, the world of dreams and intuition, the dark and watery depths of the unconscious. Throughout time the moon's luminous presence in the night sky has been an archetype of renewal and regeneration, and each phase is rife with meaning.

The new moon signifies rebirth and beginning, the crescent moon growth and creativity, the full moon intensity and illumination, and the waning moon healing and retreat. You can meditate with an intention at each phase. At the new moon, meditate to seed the beginning of a project or set in motion a desire. Drop the desire like a pebble into the waters of your psyche, and then release the outcome in trust.

The full moon is honored in all spiritual traditions—from the oldest pagan mysteries to sophisticated modern esoteric spirituality—as an optimum time for inner work. At the full moon the earth is positioned between the sun and the moon, an alignment auspicious for inner contact. Not only is the moon a visual emblem of fullness and mystery, but it pulls on the fullness of our psychic and emotional waters as well, conjuring up images of sexuality, desire, and fear. For the three days around the full moon, the gateway between the worlds is ajar, which intensifies whatever is already emerging from the unconscious. Women are especially sensitive to this pull.

Lunar rhythms directly influence ovulation and menstruation; shifting qualities of moonlight signal the pituitary to release the corresponding hormones. At the different phases of the moon, look into the night sky and let your eyes receive the light or the dark. Talk or sing to the moon, then meditate and listen, noticing the quality of your internal experience. Sleep in moonlight whenever you have the chance. Opening to the moon may help to regulate your periods, and at the very least, it's fun.

Seasonal Mysteries

The equinoxes and solstices mark the onset of each season's energy. Pagan religions honor these turning points as sacred. Most contemporary religions retain this natural wisdom, albeit cloaked behind new names. Meditate on these special days and continue throughout the season.

Spring Equinox The spring equinox occurs around March 21 (the date varies slightly, so check a calendar, and remember that folks south of the equator reverse the seasons) and marks a time to celebrate rebirth after the cold indrawing of winter. This time of equal day and night, equal light and dark, reflects a balance between the opposites, a momentary poise before the surge of summer growth. Seeds have sprouted, and we begin again with enthusiasm. Meditate with awareness of the new beginnings you are nurturing in your life. Plant some seeds as a ritual for yourself, or buy a seedling to care for. How can you fertilize and water your deepest desires?

Summer Solstice June 21 is the longest day of the year, a time to welcome the fiery sun energy of summer. Celebrate the light, power, and abundance of nature. Meditate and receive the fullness of the sun into your heart, and let its joyous energy inspire you. Expand in confidence with your own creativity, and let it too shine in the world. Throughout the summer soak up some rays (fifteen minutes daily of unscreened sunlight is recommended, in the early morning or late afternoon). Absorb the solar energy all the way to your bones; pack it into your psyche for the winter to come.

Autumn Equinox The autumn equinox arrives around September 21—another moment of parity between light and dark. This time the light of the sun is waning. "Fall" it is called, for falling leaves, and for falling back to our ground. Celebrate the harvest; acknowledge your gifts and accomplishments, however *you* define them. When we're busy, we seldom stop to appreciate what we have brought forth, the creation of our lives. At the equinox, meditate in thanks for what you've received, and continue to receive. As whispers of winter begin to tickle your inner ear, prepare for the internal gestation. Take some time for self-assessment. What is the learning? Where is the yearning?

Winter Solstice The night of December 21 is the longest night in the Northern Hemisphere. At winter solstice we enter the mystery of darkness, the journey down to the root source of being. For weeks the inklings of winter have urged us inward for silence, rest, and self-reflection. This bidding can seem incongruous amid the hurly-burly of the holidays, the commercialism and shopping panic, the frenetic festivities and sociable cheer. Unless we slow down to honor the deeper rhythm of this time, all that activity is a little crazy-making—a manic avoidance of the dark. Nonetheless, there is wisdom in these communal conventions: coming together for moral support in the long dark months and honoring the birth of the divine child, the light within, the promised return of the sun. Getting SAD (seasonal affective disorder) in the winter is indeed a hazard; we literally do need light. Sunlight is a natural antidepressant; make sure you get some (at least fifteen minutes a day). Let the thin skin of your eyelids, the backs of your knees, or your inner arms absorb the sun's rays—true nutrition for brain and bones. But in addition, heed the sacred call of winter.

Enter the dark, literally, for a solstice night meditation. Cover yourself with a blanket and lie down or sit so that you can relax completely, eyes closed. For these moments, let everything you have known drop away; let yourself die. Dwell in that emptiness and simply be. In the quietude you may hear the murmurs of your soul—its haunting, unshaped, barely audible desires. A song of yearning may fill your heart: *Remember, remember.* If an image floats into your mind, receive it. Listen well, and feel. Above all, take your time, timelessly. Hours may go by. Then, when you are ready, make a slow and gentle transition back to life. Light a candle to affirm the return of light, the eternal cycle of life. Winter solstice is nature's New Year. Receive the world with newborn eyes, new windows of the soul.

❧ MEDITATIONS

Breath as Birth and Death

Every breath recapitulates the movement of birth and death. With each inhalation we are born anew. With each exhalation, we release for an instant our tenacious hold on life and identity. Begin by focusing on one phase at a time, whichever first calls to you. Try this lying down so that you can let go more thoroughly. Make yourself completely comfortable.

The Inhalation Bring your attention to the inflow of breath. Each time you inhale, imagine that the inhalation is the first breath you have ever received. Draw in the life force, feel its creative nourishment. This may bring up memories of the first breath of your life, a sense of yourself as an infant coming into this world. For some people this is a traumatic memory; if that's true for you, use this meditation as a way to rebirth yourself with loving consciousness. What are the qualities of life you want to incarnate into? Gradually extend the length of the inhalation, taking forever to let the breath fill you in every way.

The Exhalation Bring your awareness to the outflow of breath. Imagine that each exhalation is the last breath you will ever take. Let your life force flow out with the breath; give yourself away. Release yourself completely from the particulars of your life; say good-bye to everyone and everything. As you do so you may become aware of regrets, longings, or unfinished business, or you may be filled with a poignant recognition of whom and what you truly love. Let these insights inform you about your present life. Gradually extend the length of the exhalation, taking forever to let the breath empty you out in every way.

The Complete Breath Now let your attention flow with both the inhalation and the exhalation. With each breath, imagine that you are reincarnating. You are letting go of the old life and embracing the new. Continue to breathe and feel those aspects that need to die and the qualities that need to live. Let each breath be an affirmation of awareness rooted in the deepest values of your soul.

When you feel complete with this meditation, at least for this session, make an especially careful transition back to your outer life. Open your eyes slowly and, as if newborn, simply lie there for several minutes with this fresh awareness. Then stretch gently. Know that you can return to this contemplation periodically as a way to read the inner compass for your life.

Bloodline

Meditate on the transmission of generations, your matrilineal connections back to the First Mother. All of your ancestors live on in your DNA: your mother, grandmother, and her mother before her—an unbroken lineage from the beginning of time. Feel their strength in your blood.

Begin by recognizing your womanhood, and your "wombhood." As a woman, you have a body that resonates with all women, through all of time. This commonality is in your chromosomes and in the biomorphic field of the female form.

Reflect on how you came into this life through your mother's female form, shaped by her body and blood. She, in turn, was brought forth from her mother's womb. Follow this process back through your known lineage, and then continue in your imagination all the way back to the archetypal First Mother. Imagine the first woman, in your own way; call her Eve or Lilith, or name her yourself if you like. This flow of connection is your bloodline—those who survived and lived to pass on the knowledge and strength in their genes. This is a transmission of female wisdom, a link between you and all of your ancestors.

In your DNA is the entire history of evolution, perhaps even the blueprint for the future of humanity. Ponder the intelligence and wisdom that course through your blood.

&# GOING FURTHER

Umbilicus Mundi

This is a meditation on our connection to "the Umbilicus of the World." You contemplate your navel in relation to the mythical *omphalos,* or the sacred navel of Creation. Dwelling with awareness deep in the pelvic bowl is profoundly centering and healing. Though mental pressures may pull you up and out of this connection, when you come down and in, balance is restored.

Let your attention release from your head and sink deep inside your belly. Follow your navel like a winding passageway down into the area of your womb. Breathe there for several minutes. Place your hands on your lower belly to amplify your awareness there and let yourself soften inside. (If you have had a hysterectomy, the basic energy template for the womb remains. As you rest your attention in that area, you can feel the life force there, a very healing exercise.)

Imagine that an invisible umbilical cord connects you to the Cosmic Mother, whose womb gives birth to all. Breathe from the source of life and draw its primordial nourishment in through the umbilicus into the area of your womb. You can visualize the upside-down pear shape of the uterus. What colors do you see? What color is the cord? Feel or imagine the energy circulating through your pelvis. As you exhale, send energy back out through your navel.

Acknowledge yourself as a vessel for life, not only through the literal act of childbearing but in your connection to the fecundity of nature. Breathe with the fullness and power of the belly center. Notice the sensations in the pelvis, and if emotions well up, allow them. The belly contains deep feeling and deep wisdom; somehow the two are inextricably related. Let yourself feel and dwell with it all.

Afterward, take several minutes as transition and return to a simple awareness of pleasure. Then open your eyes and gradually orient to the environment and the rest of your day.

The Chrysalis

If you are in a period of intense change in your life, meditate with the qualities of that transformation. Imagine yourself inside a chrysalis; wrap a silky, iridescent membrane around yourself and feel its soft but protective shelter. (You may want to actually wrap yourself in silk to meditate.) In the cocoon all the material for the caterpillar's transformation is contained within its own body; nothing from the outside is required. In the same way, withdraw into the chrysalis and allow your inherent wisdom to rearrange your being. Let the old form dissolve. Give over to the strange shape-changing of your metamorphosis. What new body is forming, what new wings, what new perceptions?

Be patient with yourself; this is an organic process with its own timing. Do not be too eager to emerge, but let your inner awareness and any accompanying imagery be your guide. You may well remain metaphorically within the chrysalis for months, returning to this meditation on a regular basis and allowing the imagery to change as you do. As you submit to the metamorphosis internally, be especially tender and careful with yourself in daily life. Honor the precious delicacy of this transition.

🙚 REFLECTIONS

- What insights have you discovered from exploring your rhythms?
- Most women we work with say they long for balance. What does balance mean for you?
- Take some time to recognize the qualities that are asking to be embodied at this juncture of your life. There may be a predominant tone, or two complementary rhythms. Write about them; draw or paint them. Find images from magazines that match your internal movement and create a collage, or paste them into your *Secrets* journal.

✌ SECRET #8
SAY YES TO EVERY PART OF YOURSELF

Uh-oh, I'm getting that feeling again. What is this, hormones?
Little things making me irritable, everybody looking ugly, especially myself.
I'd better snatch a meditation—I need something!

No way I can just relax. Too anxious . . .
Creepy jumpy nerves, like the whole world is crawling around
  under my skin.
Ugh. Get me outta here! Get them outta here!
Okay, okay, don't fight it; enter the sensations. Breathe . . .
Hmm, lots of energy coursing around, actually . . .
Hello! What's that crazy voice? Some new inner character?

"Grrr . . . too many, too many people . . .
Six billion bodies, wriggling and writhing all over the place.
Cars and chimneys, nuclear power plants, industrial monsters
Belching fumes from every orifice . . . Garbage and plastic everywhere—
In the streets, on the beaches, in the bellies of whales!
Rrrr, humans are so disgusting! Noxious vermin, infesting this planet . . .
Civilization? Pathetic!"

Weird. Where'd that character come from? I mean, I love humanity!
I do get, er, frustrated with all the crowding, pollution, and noise.
I have to admit, this energy is strangely compelling . . .
A sort of fierce goddess, Kali-like, wanting to protect the Earth.
Hmm, maybe it's time to donate to an environmental cause or two.
So what would satisfy this wild character? What is her meditation?

Curious . . . I hear a loud internal sound, like clashing cymbals and gongs:
Yee-ahh! Yee-ahh! What a mantra—I like it. It really matches the energy:

Fast-moving jazzy sensations, like cartoon lightning bolts
  zigzagging everywhere inside.
I'll just let those currents run through me, ride their intensity.
  Yee-ahh, Yee-ahh, Yee-ahh!

Wow. Interesting. Pure streaming now . . .
Dynamic. Energizing. Clarifying.
Let's see, can I open my eyes and stay with the sensations?
Yes . . . Ha! Makes me smile . . . a little wicked, and kind of fun.
Ah, now I feel centered, strong, and ready to go back to work.
I even sort of like people again. Who'd have thought?

  ❧ ❧ ❧

THEATER OF THE SOUL

Imagination is a wondrous capacity of being human. The body and psyche speak through metaphor, in dreams, imagery, and musings. Their poetry releases us from the tyranny of the literal, the confinement of our ordinary perception.

Women are richly complex. Behind the persona, the face we show to the world, live many other selves. When we are in touch with these other aspects, we feel more whole and life gets a lot more interesting.

C. G. Jung described the parts of the self as archetypes—perennial motifs common to all human beings. Tibetan Buddhism invokes the pantheon of benevolent and wrathful deities and visualizes them in mandalas. Artists of all kinds find images to represent the inner world. In gestalt and dream therapy you become the inner characters and let them speak. In theater a good actor accesses the cast of internal characters to expand her range of emotional expression. In every case there is an understanding that in these inner selves resides psychic energy that can be brought into consciousness and liberated for heightened creativity and vitality.

When you meditate, you experience the theater of your soul. Everybody comes onstage. The movement between different aspects of yourself is natural and necessary. It is psychic health. If we identify with just one aspect, we stop our flow. In meditation, if you have only one technique, meditation gets boring. In life, if you express only one part, your relationships become flat and you feel false. Meditation and expression are complementary. You must have a place where you can express all that is within you, so find contexts to unravel all that you feel.

A PARTY FOR ALL OF YOUR SELVES

Meditation is a meeting ground for all of your selves. During the course of a day a woman plays many roles: mother, lover, employee or boss, chauffeur, cook, maid, executive, friend, confidante, hostess, student, accountant, and life of the party. Each role represents a different way of being in the world, a different inner character with her own set of instincts and emotions. Women adeptly balance all these roles in the outer world. In meditation they show up in your inner world as well. You may as well open the door and give them all a kiss!

When you take time for yourself to meditate, any or all of these parts of yourself may come to you in turn for attention. In meditation it is as though you have come home and the kids, the dogs, the cats, the neighbors, the husband or lover, all want to come tell you about their day. Their vying for your attention is often your experience when you first close your eyes to meditate. Do not tell them to go away, just bring your attention where it is called. Having to attend to your many inner voices when you long for rest and silence may be the hardest part of meditation. But don't despair—you are on your way into relaxation.

Your inner characters show up as moods, emotions, inner dialogue, body sensations, or visual images. Let them speak. The communication may not be in words; some parts may "speak" through qualities of movement, or by suffusing you with wonderful energies, feelings, or colors. Your task is to listen, appreciate, and learn. When finally they've settled down a little bit, return to the unifying focus, which may be your breath, a sound, or a movement. By allowing your attention to flow back and forth between the focus and the inner voices, you are weaving together these disparate elements.

In the ancient language of Sanskrit, this is *yoga*, which means "linking together." Human beings are so complicated that we need to make an effort to link all our many parts together. It is part of our regular maintenance, and we suffer if we neglect this work. This linking is also *tantra*, which means "loom." You weave all elements of life—mind, body, emotions, breath, soul, individuality, and infinity—into one glorious tapestry.

DON'T MESS WITH YOUR MOODS

Allow and accept your contradictions and ever-changing moods. Don't feel you have to modify them. Meditation is not one mood, but a spacious embrace of all your moods. It is a dance between trust and mistrust, vulnerability and self-protection, boundaries and no boundaries. You may be both reverent and irreverent, or alternately rebellious and devoted. This is your nervous system doing a kind of "mood-yoga," flowing from one position to another.

You can enter meditation through any mood under the sun, or moon. Irreverence is an important mood to cultivate before and during meditation. Smash those icons, make jokes, loosen things up. Irreverence helps to free up your inner space so that you can hear your inner voices. Go ahead and talk back if you want! Piety and purity can be deadly—not in their essence, but when used to block other tones. Use your imagination. Improvise!

THE FLOW BETWEEN OPPOSITES

Life is a play of opposites, and to go in one direction you often must first go in the opposite direction. We must fall asleep to become awake; we must cry to be relieved; we must yield to healing in order to be strong. Stability comes not from remaining rigid but from constantly making fluid adjustments. During meditation we witness the swing between opposites very quickly: awareness of the inner world and awareness of the outer, expansion and contraction, pleasure and pain, safety and fear, restfulness and alertness, tension and relaxation, steady inner calm and urgency.

Between the opposites is a continuum, and that is where you live your life. Between the poles of inspiration and expiration is the continuum of breath. Between the poles of night and day is your life of work and rest. This is a celebration, not a problem. Give enough space for the opposites to fully articulate themselves. If meditation becomes boring or flat, you have been neglecting one end of the continuum. For example, you may become addicted to calmness and neglect your emotional expressiveness. Every once in a while contemplate this list:

- Diving into fantasy worlds leads to a better grip on reality.
- Losing control lets you develop greater control.
- Relaxation leads to fears and tensions coming up to be released.
- Accepting your fears and tensions leads to deeper relaxation.
- Expressing your anger and hurt leads to the possibility of forgiveness.
- Surrendering to feelings and crying leads to recovering and moving on.
- Descending into grief leads to healing and getting over it.
- Letting yourself feel the chaos leads to order.
- Surrender is power.
- Rigidity is weakness.

Opposite movements often seem conflicting or contradictory, but in truth they are complementary. Meditation is the process of turning any struggle into a dance. Opposites attract and flow toward each other: yin and yang, receptive and active, empty and full, continually moving toward and changing into each other. Much of meditation technique is about this flow and attraction. Inner balance is not a static pose but responsiveness. When you do not resist the swing between the opposites, the oscillation gives rise to a third state—integration beyond the polarities.

The opposites are in love; they need each other and cannot be fully themselves without the other. They are as inextricably entwined as the double helix in our DNA. If we get stuck in one polarity, or straddled between the two, there is no movement, we come to a kind of stalemate. So let there be flow between the mates! Here's a list of some of them:

- Individuality/Cosmic consciousness
- Will/Surrender
- Solitude/Connectedness
- Privacy/Contact
- Softness/Strength
- Selfishness/Selflessness

&8 **THE TANGO OF LIGHT AND DARK**

Marina, a healer and businesswoman, longed for connection but often felt painfully isolated. When she moved toward intimacy, powerful feelings would surface—mythic fury and shame characterized by her Greek ancestors in figures such as Medea. In our classes, Marina spiraled around this core issue, gradually realizing that by being overly peaceful and "good," she had submerged her wildness. Through movement, she found a creative way to release the tremendous energy, and her inner struggle between light and dark became a passionate tango.

"I'm falling in love . . . with hate. Rage surges from my guts every time I reach out toward life. Such a fine line between love and hate—if I can only hold that edge in between . . ." Her challenge was "letting go but not losing myself in the process—playing that edge. This was my initiation, changing the course of my destiny. No longer half-alive, half-dead, I am choosing to fully live."

Marina now emits a womanly power and clarity. Though moving with the inner currents of passion will need to be an ongoing practice, "something opened in me, I don't feel the same. My heart opened, and I look at people through softer eyes." Embracing hate has liberated her love.

- Saying yes/Saying no
- Dependence/Independence
- Attraction/Aversion
- Wisdom/Innocence
- Passion/Peace

Complementary tones can support your primary role in life. Do meditations that enhance your dominant mode as well as its opposite. For example:

- If you are a warrior, foster both strengthening and softening.
- If you are a caregiver, foster both compassion for others and self-nourishing.
- If you are an artist, foster both intensity and equanimity.
- If you are a mother, foster both holding and letting go.

INNER ALLIES

If you identify which of your inner parts is calling you, giving it attention will make your meditation deeper. A self you do not know very well may emerge to be the goddess of meditation for a day, for a month, or for years. Your guide may be your magical child, or the wise person in you, or your dancer self you gave up when you had babies, or the wild and free hellion you were in college. You never know which archetype may be your ally in meditation. The "killer bitch" may be the only one who can tear you away from the needs of others and say, "I am going to meditate now. Let the world turn without me for a while."

Welcome all your selves to the party. Let them come as they are. Let the naughty, mischievous, contrary parts have their say. Even the so-called negative voices bestow secret blessings when you listen to them.

The rules of meditation are different from the conventions of social interaction: you accept and explore everything. As you get used to meditation, you will trust the relaxation and safety of meditation to be strong enough to contain *anything* that rises up to be expressed. A difficult emotion or character may become your strongest ally. Let it share its desires, its fears, its way of seeing the world. These can be messages to you of what is missing in your life.

The Utterly Simple Principle

Go with what is, but participate consciously.

In every meditation, ask yourself: What does the energy want? Then find the way to respond. When a difficult mood, character, or emotion has you in its grip, you have a choice, an aesthetic choice, depending on the texture and quality that you want to cultivate in that moment. You can meditate with pleasure to soothe and nourish yourself, assuaging the emotional tension. Sometimes that satisfies the inner call, as long as you do not judge or deny what's going on.

Your other choice is to enter the energy more fully and take it on. Sometimes the inner character or mood is so persistent that the only way out is in. Join it, become it, learn from it. This is a courageous path, and not for everyone all the time, but it is very freeing and integrative.

Wise Elder, Wild Child

Within each woman is a sacred triad: the child-self, the everyday-self, and the wise woman. These three levels exist simultaneously as concentric spheres of awareness that enfold and inform one another.

The woman you are today has the capacity to wrap her arms of consciousness around your young and tender inner self. You can hear the needs and desires of the child within and nurture her. In the same way the wise woman is always present in your psyche, always holding and caring for you. Whether you imagine her as the elder you will become or as the archetypal Grandmother or Great Mother, she is eternally with you, patiently waiting for you to ask of her wisdom.

In any meditation you can tune in to these inner allies. Each carries a key to your joy, knowledge, and peace. There will be times when you feel about five years old inside—whiny, fragile, dependent, unruly, or wild. This is the time for your adult self to hold, soothe, and heed the child within. If you do not, she will only cry, scream, or flail more loudly until you respond. In your inner world, gather her into your arms, if she will let you. If she has been neglected (if you have been neglected), she may be hiding behind a rock all covered in mud or up in a tree staring at you with wary eyes and twigs in her hair. If so, simply be present, and let her know you will not abandon her again. Eventually she will begin to trust and will take you into her magical world. This is a commitment, ultimately to yourself, so be prepared to follow through. No matter what your age, you must tend to her often throughout the rest of your life.

Then there will be times when it is your everyday self who needs to be held by an older and wiser loving consciousness. You are tired from caring for everyone else, from working hard and holding the world together. You cannot muster the physical or mental strength to do one more thing. You are depressed or confused or overwhelmed. This is the moment to call upon the Wise One. With your inner voice, ask her to appear and allow the image to unfold. Let her show you to her cave at the center of the earth, or follow the trail to her cabin in the woods. She may speak in words or visions, hand you sacred talismans, or communicate simply with her silent being. She may hold you to her breast, rock you in her lap, and sing. Lean back into her wide embrace, breathe, release, and receive.

There is a mystic truth in the phrase "to be in touch" with parts of the self. Stay in touch inside. Envision your child-self held by you held by your wise woman self, all three in harmonious rapport. To experience the unity of this inner trinity is a profound revelation and sustenance for the soul.

Shadow Self

Ponder on this: when embraced and transmuted with consciousness, Sloth, Gluttony, Avarice, Wrath, Envy, Lust, and Pride are lively—the Seven Lively Sins.

The more conscious you are of your shadow, the less it will be acted out unconsciously and damage your relationships. Locked within shadow energy is tremendous libido, or life force, waiting to be channeled. When the darker impulses are denied and forced underground, the inner war creates all kinds of havoc. Because the psyche always seeks balance, it will attempt to heal the split by bringing to awareness what has been repressed—one way or the other.

A hint on identifying your shadow: the very qualities that you hate in others tend to exist in yourself—in spades. Feeling that you are righteous and justified is always a clue, and if unacknowledged, this will manifest as unwitting cruelty to others—often those closest to you, or as internalized cruelty to yourself. The more you disown your shadow and turn away, the bigger it grows, tagging along right behind you, ever more malodorous and dank. There is no getting rid of it, and the closer someone gets to you, the more obvious the shadow pattern becomes. Shadow energy is quite magnetic and unerringly draws in the perfect relationships to dramatize and liberate itself. Sooner or later you have to turn around, face yourself, and learn to dance with the dark.

One of the great challenges of meditation is to tolerate the self-knowledge and inevitable insights of conscience. When you meditate, you can get a whiff of what needs to be addressed before it sneaks out inappropriately somewhere in your life. Or if it has already done some harm, you can meditate and track back to the original purpose behind the impulse. Welcome the messenger; don't kill her.

Half your meditation might be a fantasy of punching somebody out. Kate, a black woman attorney, professor, and advocate for gender and racial equality, was shocked when this happened after she had experienced weeks of pleasure and peace in meditation. Since her personality is gentle and conscientious and doesn't include "the bitch," aggression and revenge were shadow qualities for her. She is a beautiful and brilliant woman, so other people are often envious of her. When she found out she'd been betrayed by a female colleague, she was flooded with images of telling the woman off. In the fantasy she was slapping and kicking her colleague, and she could feel power surging in her body. This was her nervous system practicing the integration of disowned energy. Her meditation now includes, "I give thanks that there is a part of me, an instinct inside me, that is willing to stand up for me and fight for myself, to protect me. I give thanks for this energy rising in me."

To feel shadow power can bring up a combination of joy and sorrow. Don't be afraid of the sorrow. It's the melting away of the old feelings. And don't hold back from the joy—you deserve it.

Warrior Spirit

One archetype that can be an especially powerful ally for women today is the female warrior—aggressive, strong in body and spirit, able to meet any challenge that comes her way.

Aggression can be healthy and necessary. You can be aggressive when called for, even if you are peaceful and harmonious inside. The purpose of the peacefulness and compassion that meditation engenders is not to domesticate you or to make you passive. There is an instinctive part of every person whose role is protection of self and others. We need her.

Women warriors pop up occasionally in popular fiction. Current favorites are the TV characters "Xena, Warrior Princess" and "La Femme Nikita"—women who are physically and mentally honed, a little wild, full-bodied, gutsy, and lethal if necessary. But notice that these fantasy females still embody soul; they make their choices from the heart. That's why we love them.

Women must stay connected with their primal, raw energy, their natural aggression. This is a key to your life force, your health, and your power. Without access to that energy, you are too easily the victim, too readily submissive and subservient; without it, something inside you shrivels and dies. Anger is a signal of this healthy aggression trying to protect you; behind the anger is vital energy that can set you free. Aggression is the same life force that causes a new shoot of grass to push up through the soil, even through cement, to seek the light. If you suppress that aggression, you suppress the natural movement of expansion that is absolutely necessary for your health—mental, emotional, and physical. We've seen so many women who, after reclaiming this energy, have gone from pale, bloodless versions of themselves to women thriving with vitality and joy.

Women warriors are not just fictional. Throughout history female warriors have been just as fierce and brutal as their male counterparts, if not more so. What is fictional is the notion that women are exclusively and by nature passive, peaceful, and pleasing. The Greeks gave us the word *Amazon,* virtually synonymous with "woman warrior." It means "one-breasted": Amazons allegedly cut off their own right breast, the better to shoot their arrows. Talk about commitment! These figures may well have been mythical, a male invention symbolic of their fear of feminine power. Likewise, the existence of such women in South America is questionable; they were reputedly seen by Spanish explorers, who thus gave the river its name. However, the 1995 excavation of sites dating from 600 B.C. to 300 A.D. in Pokrovka, Russia, revealed the remains of numerous women buried with weapons. Marco Polo wrote about warrior horsewomen during his travels in Mongolia, noting that one princess amassed a great fortune by wrestling and vanquishing her many suitors—who each gambled and lost one hundred horses to her. (She never did marry.) The celebrated Celtic queen Bodicea raised an army of women and men in bloodthirsty retaliation against the Romans. In Dahomey, Africa, women were until quite recently honored as ferocious warriors on behalf of their tribe.

Not a dainty picture of our sex. Our reasons for aggression may differ from men's reasons, but women in righteous revenge can be merciless, savage, and cruel. If we can admit this, we might heal a serious rift between the sexes. Violence is a female attribute too; no longer can we simply blame the Other.

Meditation can help us to claim our warrior energy—and to *mediate* it with self-reflection. We can clarify our beliefs so that we act on them with dignity, strength, and understanding. Obviously women today don't have to take up arms literally. But many of us take up the sword for such causes as the environment, global consciousness, and compassionate communication. Becoming strong advocates of relational, life-affirming values is perhaps the best contemporary expression of this female warrior spirit.

EMOTIONAL SAVVY

A resilient, well-lubricated emotional body promotes a rich inner life and deeper intimacy in our outer life. Access to our emotional depths gives us the resilience to live in the world with courage, sensitivity, and gusto.

Emotions are adaptive. They inform us of our basic instincts that keep us safe and thriving. They feed our intuition—our "truthsense," which relies on awakened sensibilities for accurate perception. They foster empathy and compassion—essential for personal and global peace—which depend on a refined understanding of ourselves and others. Because of these expanded perceptions, "emotional intelligence" is gaining acknowledgment as equal in value to cerebral intelligence. The more inclusive our emotional range, the broader our perceptual ability. It thus behooves us all to cultivate a full spectrum of emotion.

As women, we arguably have a head start on emotional intelligence, and most of us honor this native skill. A female approach to meditation can and must include the conscious exercise of this capacity to feel. What could be more obvious? Yet many people believe that emotions are obstacles to enlightenment, the reactions of an impure "ego," and a sure sign of failure in meditation. In the name of spirituality powerful emotions are subtly shunned, like the village madwoman, as far too messy, unpredictable, dangerous, and distracting.

Granted, all of us want a surcease now and then from the intensity of what we feel, and it is good to have some meditations in our repertoire that serve that function. (Check out "Secret #9: Rest in Simplicity.") Most of the time, however, emotions show up for a good reason: something needs to move within us and needs to be communicated, at least to ourselves. Stifling emotions only leads to fragmentation, especially for women. We therefore advocate the radical exploration of the movement of emotion, untidy as this may seem.

The realm of emotion can indeed be a tricky, sticky wicket, and finding balance is quite an art. Everybody knows people who are "out of control," affecting and infecting everyone around them. Classically, women are given a hellish choice in dealing with volatile emotion: confined to either repression or acting out, they can choose to damage themselves or to damage others. All of us have observed women who are stuck in one extreme or the other: the muted, self-punishing state of holding back feelings, or the manipulative, hysterical, blaming style of expressing them. Either way, such women seem controlled by emotion—who wants that? Yet almost every woman finds herself gravitating to one end of the spectrum or the other.

If your mother, for example, suffered in one of these modes, you may have decided to become the opposite. If she was withdrawn and withholding, you probably make damn sure you don't hold anything in;

the Drama Queen may be one of your favorite parts. In the opposite scenario, if she was overwhelming in some way, you may be an expert at keeping yourself under wraps; the Control Freak may be a familiar, comfortable role. Or maybe you've had it with the mushy, sloppy, sappy style of all those femmes who "just really, really feel that way," so you've turned away from emotionalism in disgust.

Detachment can be an occupational hazard. Caretakers may desperately crave an emotional moratorium; saturated by others' needs, they're too tired to take care of their own. Women executives exert tremendous self-control to succeed in the male-dominated business world; retrieving their softer sensibilities may threaten their status quo. One of our friends, an ob/gyn, is immersed all day in the gushes of female emotion and bodily fluids. The last thing Terri wants is more gushiness! Yet she longs for the honesty and intimacy of her own emotional expressiveness. What to do? How do we allow the fullness of what must be felt without suppression, obsession, or possession?

There are many forms of psychotherapy that explore the content of emotion, your personal history, and its effect on your present life. The mental deconstruction of emotion can elucidate reaction patterns that no longer serve you. You can learn to identify and express your truthful response. This is extremely helpful in coming to terms with painful experiences that every human being undergoes, and we recommend any technique of befriending difficult feelings that appeals to you.

Beware, however, of talking yourself out of the deeper gift of emotion. Here's the secret: there is another mode entirely, the delicate art and skill of consciously riding the emotion back to its primal source.

In meditation you can get "underneath" the content—the story, memory, image, or event attached to the feeling. We do not mean dissociation or detachment, or even "mindfulness." Behind the mask of each character, behind the label of each emotion, is pure life force. The emotion itself is a sign of some essential energy that wants to circulate through your system, a palpable, physical stream of power. Whatever the emotion, you can enter and ride its current in meditation. You can consciously join with the stream and let it inform you.

When you suppress your vital energy, it has dire consequences for your physical and emotional well-being. When life force backs up, it is experienced as:

- Irritability
- Depression
- Tiredness
- Confusion
- Moodiness
- Headaches
- Symptoms of illness

These conditions often arise from an injunction against some quality of expression. An emotion is a powerful surge of energy that, once activated, must be fulfilled somehow. Waves don't just stop or go away. If suppressed, emotional energy becomes a real troublemaker—stagnating in the body, creating mental imbalance, or sneaking out irrepressibly at the most awkward times, usually with a vengeance.

If you suspect that energy is jammed up inside you, ask yourself what might be hiding. What feeling or inner character would be especially unacceptable right now? Remember, the more taboo the expression, the greater the psychic energy to be liberated. If an inner character or emotion has been rejected, sent into isolation in the shadows of your internal world, it's probably festering with the need to come out. In meditation you can welcome it back into circulation. Give it refuge, bring it into your sanctuary, and get to know it. Feel its life force and receive its gift.

An excruciating vulnerability may be asking for acceptance, or perhaps some volatile, politically incorrect attitude or dark rage lurking in your heart is demanding to be recognized. The feeling may be so unsocialized, primitive, or preverbal that your only clue is an inchoate sadness or vague irritation. No matter what the emotion, it is extremely important to accept and give over to it, in the safety of your meditation. Your practice is *not* about acting out inappropriately, but it *is* about allowing that tone of energy to move through you fully—consciously.

Let's take the example of anger, so crucial yet problematic. People who identify themselves as spiritual, especially women, typically have a tenacious taboo against anger. They will do every meditative practice they know to block it out: being compassionate, surrendering, washing themselves with white light. By whitewashing the anger, they cheat themselves of the gift of its primal force and the honesty it reveals. They lose the footing necessary to mobilize themselves in their lives and can wander in disempowered confusion for years.

Say you sit down to meditate and notice that you're a little out of sorts. You begin to focus on your breath, or a mantra, and like a good girl try to drown out the irritation. It persists. You find yourself thinking of some past or present situation and discover, uh-oh, you're angry. Ordinarily you might think, *I shouldn't be angry. I should forgive. I understand. I'm a loving person.* If you investigate the anger, however, you will undoubtedly see through the dynamics of that situation to greater clarity about what needs to be expressed. Something didn't get to move in that situation and is still waiting to be released. Now, here's the real skill: you can also allow the fiery quality of anger to surge through you. Let it dance inside. Let the flame expand and charge your whole aura. These sensations become your meditative focus. The physical sense of yourself as energy will become heightened as you harness the force and let it vitalize you. This awareness creates more personal space and reclaims the strength to deal with that person or event most effectively. Then, after meditation, you have more choice in how you actually respond to situations that make you angry, neither repressing nor misusing your anger.

On the other hand, some women get bound up in righteous blame. If anger or resentment is a habitual response for you, a familiar style of handling discomfort, the message may be to delve beneath it. Perhaps your reactivity threatens your relationships or the health of your heart. Dare to enter the deeper emotion that is calling—probably something that makes you feel vulnerable, like sadness or fear. Let yourself soften. Tolerate the sensations as your chest and heart relax. To enter the tenderness may feel like a fate worse than death, but it opens you to the depth of connection you crave. A new compassion for yourself and others will undoubtedly emerge.

When powerful emotions surface, people are often afraid that they will get stuck in them, that the grief or rage or fear will never end. But emotions are very fluid; when you accept them and let them flow without resistance, they can change quickly. Anger turns to joy, sorrow turns to love, fear turns to anger or excitement. The movement itself becomes a joyful release. This ever-changing energy flow is both the challenge and the ecstasy of awareness.

The fluidity of a woman's nature can be difficult to manage. Lorin often jokes about how a woman experiences more emotional fluctuations in one day than a man does in an entire year! It is thus especially necessary for us to consciously navigate within the flux; because we are emotionally more labile, it's a must that we "stay current" with ourselves. No, *labile* is not related to *labia* (too bad—a completely different etymology); it means "open to change, adaptable"—thank you very much! When you learn to ride the currents of emotion, you will have a new-found experience of integration, a tangible sense of power and relief. It can change your life. Adopt a new motto: "Labile and Loving It!"

Your Full Spectrum

Each feeling tone or inner character is like a color in your palette to enjoy and use creatively, and you become more aware of this the more you explore. Let your meditation endorse and exercise your full spectrum—from ultraviolet to infrared, from exquisitely refined sensitivity to the deep raw heat of passion.

Develop an appreciation of your personal aesthetic, your individual tones. Maybe your palette favors subtle, delicately shaded pastels, or maybe intensely vibrant, electric hues are more your style. Your embodiment of each energetic color, your "blue" or "red," has nuances different from anyone else's. This is life expressing itself through you, in the particular way it can do so only through you.

At the center of your color wheel *you* reside in awareness. As you free up each emotional tone, the wheel begins to spin, and the colors swirl all around you. Within the swirling sphere of color the entire spectrum of emotion circulates all around—the free play of primal energy. Any emotional color is available to you at any moment, as you should need. Imagine that you are standing at the center, harnessing and absorbing the movement of that vital force. This is the mastery, the art and skill of emotional balance: staying centered in the full spectrum of movement—Shakti's timeless, blissful dance.

🙠 EXPLORATIONS

- What are your familiar moods or emotions? Notice the alternation of moods in a meditation (for example, anxious, irritable, bored, playful, mischievous, sarcastic, fearful, buoyant, peaceful, ecstatic)
- Lover, Mother-Nurturer, Child-self, Warrior, Martyr, Priestess, Hermit, Sorceress-Bruja-Witch, Curandera-Healer, Ancient Crone-

Wise Woman, Fool, Bitch, Slut, Madonna, Whore—these arche-types are ways to describe how energy expresses itself in the psyche. How many of them can you identify in your psyche? Which are your strongest? Which is most secret?

- Where do you get glimpses of your power?
- What fictional or historical characters do you identify with?
- What mythical beings intrigue you (for example, dragons, elves, angels, devas, fairies, unicorns, demons, monsters, gorgons)? What qualities do they offer?
- Which energies or archetypes scare you? Why?

🐝 WARM-UP: PUT YOUR MIND ON THE FLOOR

Sometimes we cannot do justice to our inner voices by simply writing in a journal. Here is a technique to use once in a while. First, keep track of the background chatter of your mind for a few days, enough to get a page of dialogue. Put this in a journal or wherever you feel like writing it. You might carry around some scraps of paper at all times so you can jot down everything you hear.

Then transfer the sentences to index cards, three-by-five or five-by-eight, whichever size you prefer to work with. Write down one thought per card. Lay the cards out in an array of any kind. Give your thoughts plenty of room. Do you need even more space? Similar thoughts can be put closer together, and dissimilar ones can be put further away. Then sit in the middle, with 360-degree awareness, and acknowledge each one. Your inner thoughts may be completely startled to even be noticed.

Look at each card and consider what its message is. Spend a minute with each one. Think of all the lines of dialogue and the feelings it gives you. Then switch and look at another. Notice asymmetries. What are the imbalances? If there is a critical voice, is there also a supportive voice? If there is a voice calling you to duty, is there a voice calling you to rest and recharge? If there is a voice warning you not to get involved with one person, is there a voice encouraging you to spend more time with your friends?

There is no reason to stick with words. You could go to a toy store or garage sale and buy action figures—Wonder Woman, a medieval princess, and so on. Use them. Or you could use drawings, swatches of clothes, colors, or symbolic objects. The Motherpeace tarot is a wonderful, woman-savvy deck with interesting paintings and symbols on round cards. You could get statues of saints and arrange them. Each saint has a different personality, a different message. Or statues of gods and goddesses. You can tell which images are working for you because they seem to become enchanted. When children are playing, the string or doll they are holding has life to it. Your cards or dolls will have life to you for a moment. An exercise such as this is a form of play. Play is not just for kids.

When you are done, put your figures or cards back in the box. Honor each one, because you will undoubtedly continue to learn from it. Now the thoughts aren't just inside your head—they are outside, with much more room in which to operate. After doing this, you may notice that the thoughts don't crowd you as much when you are meditating.

- Identify the images that appear in your dreams or fantasies, or the ones you are attracted to in art, theater, dance, photographs, or movies.
- Create a collage of inner characters from images you find in magazines or that you paint.

&8 SKILL CIRCLE #8:
HOW TO MEDITATE WITH
YOUR INNER THEATER

In this section we introduce some methods of working with your inner characters and emotions. Accept the complexity of your meditative experience. Behind every role we play is an internal character, and behind each character is an emotion. You can enter your inner theater from any one of these.

Celebrate your inner characters. Together they make up the whole community that is you. Each represents a different type of intelligence, and each has a different take on any situation. This lets you see things from new angles. Let them all come into the circle so they can give their gift to the community. Transformation comes when we embrace all our energies and let them speak, dance, and sing together.

Emotions

The emotional body circulates the full spectrum of emotional color, and any experience is usually a complex mélange of more than one. A particular mood or feeling may come to the foreground at any moment but, when acknowledged, changes into or is joined by another.

Whatever the emotion, you can track it in meditation. The motion of each emotion varies with the individual, but generally it can be upward (glee, delight, laughter), downward (sinking feelings, sadness, depression), inward (shame, dread, envy), or outward (anger, blame, joy, adoration). Some of the sensations associated with the emotions are fiery and expansive (anger), sinking and melting down (sadness), warmth and inner glow (love), tightness and contraction (fear), trembling and restlessness (anxiety), and effervescence (joy).

In addition, each emotion may have an image. It is very helpful to give these energies creative form, especially the more uncomfortable ones. The image itself is a container that gives you a creative way to relate to the emotion without becoming overly "identified" with it or possessed by it. That is why we recommend that you discern which of your inner characters is expressing the feeling. Then you can employ any of the methods we detail here to access the gift of energy.

If you are experiencing emotional stagnation, you may require some assistance to get back in the flow. The most effective healing techniques operate on this wisdom and should always lead you back to your own empowered participation rather than foster dependency. By all means, seek counseling or therapy if the emotions seem overwhelming or unmanageable.

Inner Characters

Through the "Explorations" you have identified some of your inner characters. When you meditate, you will often be visited by one of them; someone will sneak out from the wings and show up on center stage demanding an audience. Each character always brings a gift.

Because the inner world speaks in symbols, imagery, and metaphors, you need to free yourself from the bounds of literal reality. Your inner character may do or say things that are physically impossible or morally inappropriate. That does not matter; what matters is the quality of the energy that is seeking acknowledgment. What you choose to do with the information—how you express it in your relationships—comes later. For now, let your imagination take flight.

Welcome the character onto the stage. What face do you see? What kind of voice do you hear, and what is it saying? How is it costumed? What is it doing, and how does it move? What energy does this character represent?

Sometimes the character appears as a feeling without a face or image, but you can track the sensations. What is the quality of energy, and what does it want? Does it want you to hide, or does it want you to break free? Does it want lots of space, or would it rather be cozy and snug? Does it want to buzz and tingle through your body, or does it want to soothe your nerves? Is it trying to get you to take action, or to avoid it? Does it want you to whisper nonsense syllables, sing at the top of your lungs, or spin a long tale of woe? Do you feel like crying, laughing, sneering, spitting, cooing, drooling, panting, moaning, or raging? Do you want to send energy out of your body, or draw it in?

Whether you are working with a specific image or not, here are a few more ways to explore and flesh out your inner character.

Find the Gesture Begin to hunt for a movement or gesture that feels satisfying—anything at all. The inner image may demonstrate the movement for you, or you can play around and let your body discover it by surprise. You may find yourself curled up in a tight little ball, or furiously stabbing at the air. Your hands may be drawn to your heart, or pulled into a reach of longing and passion. You may feel like running away, jumping up and down, quaking like an aspen leaf, or standing still like a mountain. When you find the movement, or series of movements, it will show you graphically what the energy is about.

Repeat the gesture over and over and let it change in any way. How does your breath flow in the movement? Does a sound want to come? Give over to the energy until it seems completely satisfied. Then bring it to a pause and track the inner sensations even more deeply. This can take you into meditation again, or into writing from your experience.

Dialogue Before or after moving with the energy, you can have a conversation with the character. Your ego-self can ask questions and listen to the response. One way to do this is by writing in your journal. You can begin with the question "What do you want?" and then allow your pen to flow with the answer. When the response is moving, strange or shocking, it's a pretty good clue that you are tapping in to a hidden truth.

Spontaneous Writing As you meditate, or immediately after moving, invite one word to float into your awareness that hints at the energy of the character. It can appear instantly, or you may need to wait for it to drift in. Again, the word can be anything, and it may very well be surprising or odd. Then go to your journal and write that one word on your page. Let any associations come and let them flow out through your pen. If you have been dancing with the energy, that dance is still in your body and the quality of movement can gurgle, spurt, or stream its way onto the paper. Don't even try to be logical, make sense, or construct complete sentences. This is a time to wedge open the rational constructs and be as nonsensical as possible so that the truth of your psyche can poke up through the cracks. Keep writing any words that come. If you get stuck, repeat the words you just wrote over and over until they finally shift and shape-change into something new.

After about five minutes of writing, stop and read what has come through. Then, if you have time, you can meditate or move again with those impressions.

Witnessing Sometimes the characters want to be witnessed by other human beings. It is very freeing to have another person hold the conscious attention while you enter and let go into the expression. A trusted friend or group, a therapist, or a class can be a wonderful context in which to bring the energy out of isolation and into communication.

❧ MEDITATIONS

The Pendulum

This meditation facilitates the flow between the opposites (see the list of complementary tones on page 174). You can also choose two inner parts that appear to be at odds.

Completely give in to one pole of the continuum, one of your opposites. Then completely give in to its complement. Give over to the intensity of your full range of expression. Become each quality without reservation—no postmodern irony, no modulation. For example, for five minutes be a tyrannical boss who is going to stay on the project until it is done, driving everyone to exhaustion in the process. Then for another five minutes enter into the feeling: *I am going to leave it all. I don't care.*

The key is to rest in the pure tone of each; go all the way into the state without holding back. Holding back throws us off balance and prevents life and the body from flowing between opposites. In life situations it may not be appropriate to express the full intensity, but in meditation you can.

Let your attention swing back and forth a few times between the two modes of expression. As it does, know that you are weaving together the various aspects of your being. Consider this your inner yoga.

Jazz Breath

This breath is very enlivening and fun. Add it to your sitting meditation, or take it into movement.

Bring your attention to your breath and begin to focus on the exhalation. Let your mouth open and hear the whispering sound of breath flow out. In this case we're going for the aspirated sound rather than using your vocal cords. Explore different breath sounds: *shh, huuu, sssss, chah*. Does anybody remember Jimmy Durante? He was famous for his "Ha cha cha!"

Now get interested in the rhythm of the exhalation and begin to play with the breath sound like your own jazz riff. You can even do this to percussive music and change rhythms to match some of its beats, as though you're part of the band. As you get more involved with this expression, you may happen upon a compelling energy or inner character. If so, go for it—let the energy have free rein. This breath can naturally lead to movement, so dance those rhythms too. Have a blast!

By breathing expressively this way, you are freeing up the energy of your solar plexus. As your diaphragm and lungs pump life force through your body, the muscles all through your belly and chest are engaged and released. This is a powerful cleansing and energizing for all of your internal organs. The solar plexus is generally associated with personal power, as well as the ability to receive information from your environment. You don't have to force or tighten your belly. Don't hyperventilate; just breathe in a free and playful way.

After a few minutes of this, let the intentional breathing subside. Allow the breath be whatever it wants to be and simply notice the aftereffects. You may feel more awake. Your skin may tingle, or perhaps a sense of vital energy is coursing through your whole body. It is good to do a couple of rounds of the breathing and stillness. When you feel ready, begin again. Each time opens up new discoveries.

❧ GOING FURTHER

Behind the Mask

Everybody has a persona we show to the world, a familiar and safe identity that we let others see. The word *persona* originated in ancient theater and refers to the masks that the actors wore to represent the different characters. Behind the persona or mask that you usually wear is a complex human being with many inner parts. In my "Moving Theater" workshops I like to say, "Identity is highly overrated." By this I mean that when people speak of "finding themselves," they think of the self as a thing, a fixed identity rather than a rich range of movement between many ever-changing parts. This exercise brings movement to your mask to elicit some of these other selves.

You can do this before meditation to free yourself up, or you can do it in conjunction with "Jazz Breath" or "What a Character!" Begin in a comfortable position and take a few minutes just to bring awareness to your face. Don't change anything yet; simply observe. Notice the sensations and expressions in your mouth, eyes, and eyebrows. How tight are your lips and jaw? What's happening with your tongue? Is there tension in the muscles around your eyes and forehead? What are the sensations around your nose and cheeks? If you saw yourself in a mirror right now, what feeling would you see?

Now bring your attention to the inside of your mouth, the space inside. Very gently and easily, begin to let your mouth change shape: separate your teeth, lightly pucker your lips, move your tongue around. Then slightly wiggle your eyebrows and let your eyes take on expression. Feel little movements in your cheeks and nostrils.

Notice how every new movement opens up a kind of expression. Start to play with these qualities. Smile, grimace, pout, stick out your tongue, frown, open your mouth wide. You'll probably find that your breath rhythm changes as you play through the face, so let it take on expressiveness too. Let some sounds escape. The movement may be very dramatic, like Balinese masks, but it does not have to be. In fact, the smallest nuances can take you into the most profound feelings and subtleties of character. Slow down and see how minimal the movement can be.

After several minutes of this, pause and feel. Observe the sensations through your face, the tingle and liveliness on your skin, the alertness in your eyes. If emotions or associations have been stirred up, let them move through you. Take them into meditation or write in your journal. Welcome the feelings and any image from your inner theater.

What a Character!

Sometimes an inner character just shows up when you close your eyes and tune in to your inner world. As described in the skill circle, you can meditate with its energy. Each character is a multifaceted experience; go with whatever impression presents itself to you—an emotion, a body sensation, a visual image, a longing or desire. Maybe the character announces its presence in words: "Hold me!" or, "Get me out of here!" or, "I don't give a damn!" Get curious, listen, and explore.

Sometimes you may want to invite a particular character into your meditation. Elicit your "alter egos" to access their quality of energy: the Woman Warrior, the Wise Elder, the Wildwoman, or the Beast. Any of the characters you identified in the "Explorations" can come into play.

Take plenty of time in your sitting meditation to explore the sensory details and to let the quality of energy run through your body.

In addition, you can dance as the inner character. Each aspect of your psyche has a distinct energy, and thus a different body and way of moving. Tune in to the qualities and emotions it expresses. What is its dance? Join that movement. What music would match the feeling? Put on music that supports this quality, breathe with the feeling, and let your body become the body of the emotion or character.

Experiment with alternating between dancing and meditating. Each mode amplifies the other, so give yourself plenty of time to explore both.

Yakitty-Yak, You Can Talk Back

There are many ways to relate to the inner voices. Try this one if you want to practice irreverence. When your mind is very noisy, identify several of the voices and start to talk back. You can direct them, like a movie director. "Okay, you over there, Big Ogre, go over there to the corner and hold up the walls. Thank you very much." Or if you're in the mood to exercise your tyrannical power, "coach" them as if you were a demanding sports coach, Marine Corps drill instructor, or some other kind of coach. To see models of this kind of character, you can rent a movie that features a coach or DI, such as *GI Jane, Any Given Sunday,* or *An Officer and a Gentleman.*

For example, if you have a critical voice saying, "You aren't doing enough. Your work is inadequate," you could respond, "You call that a critical voice? Ha! You are pathetic. Put more *oomph* into it! Flog me with your scorn! Oh, you can't, eh? You're not so tough after all!" If it is a fearful voice telling you the world is scary ("Watch out when you walk down the street," "Don't take any risks"), then talk back and say, "You call that something to be scared of? What about the end of the universe? What about a meteor hitting earth? What's the matter with you? Have you no imagination? Some horror movie writer you'd make! Why don't you just slink off and hide your head in shame?"

Talk back to at least two of the voices you have mapped. If a voice is silent, you can tease it for being silent. "What, you don't have anything to say today? Cat got your tongue?"

This exercise is one way to own your shadow qualities. Notice how it feels to be able to talk back to tyrannical voices. Steal their power back by admitting and utilizing your own.

❧ REFLECTIONS

- Which energies do you find the most familiar? Which are most difficult to accept? Sooner or later you will need to befriend a full gamut of internal tonalities. When you are ready, approach them, talk with them, or let them approach you. Often the strangest energies have the most important teaching.

- Do you sense that something is missing from your life? What inner character is calling you? Does it speak with a whisper, cry, giggle, or shout? What area of your life is it concerned about? How can you honor its wisdom or satisfy its desire?

- What quality of expression are you ready to say yes to? What taboos are you ready to dare?

- If you honor your complexity, the simplicity of your essence will emerge. The voices will quiet, because you have listened to them all. They will become quieter not because of repression but because they know they have been heard.

- Learn to be sensitive to the call of an inner character. Let its spirit flow through you and inform you. Let it find expression in some way. Use dance, painting, and intuitive writing to free up your energy. Then meditate to center the energy and reclaim it for your life.

- Bring more expression into your relationships. For example, Lorin and I often improvise around the house. Some inner voice comes up in one of us, and we let it speak, in "quotes." We get into hilarious skits. This improv helps to diffuse little irritations when they sometimes come up between us. Pretty handy, eh?

SECRET #9
REST IN SIMPLICITY

Everything is so complicated. Decisions to make, problems to solve.
A million thoughts, a thousand different feelings. . . .
I'm losing it! Okay, I admit it—I'm overwhelmed.
Usually I can keep things under control, make things happen.
Why can't I now? Maybe if I just try a little harder . . .
Ugh, I think I have to lie down.

Just a couple of minutes, then I'll get back on my horse.
Down to the floor, put my belly to the ground. Ah, that's better.
Let the big belly of the Earth hold everything for me for a while.
But . . . who am I if I'm not the one who organizes everything,
Who holds the myriad threads in her mind and keeps track of it all?
Will I just dissolve, like the Wicked Witch?
Well, I guess I can afford to let go for, uh . . . five or ten minutes . . .

Breathe . . . yes, just breathe (huge inhalation).
Containing everybody else can really wear you out.
Maybe I need to be contained. You know what would be great?
If somebody heavy would just lie on top of me, hold me down, calm me.
Or if I could be completely surrounded by earth substance . . .
That's it, I'll imagine I'm part of the ground,
Just sink right down—solid, weighty, slow . . .
(huge exhalation).

Whoa, where am I? That was more than ten minutes!
Let's see if I can even move. My bones are so relaxed . . .
Yep, there are my fingers, my toes.
There's my breath—still here, taking care of itself just fine.

What if I try to open my eyes? Roll over, look around . . . oops, slowly . . .
Hmm, it's a new world out there. Everything looks so fresh . . .
It's a new world in here too. Sort of . . . newborn. Connected, held, safe.

Now, make my way back to my chair . . . sit here for a minute or two . . .
Ah. I see it now. All this stuff will get sorted out, in time . . .
Yes, all in good time . . .

&⅊ &⅊ &⅊

SERENITY

Sometimes we *crave* simplicity. We want to unplug from the demands of our lives, from everything requiring our attention. At such times meditation can be a breath of fresh air.

We all know the desire to be held by something larger than ourselves. We want to be taken care of, to be the child in the Mother's arms, to be protected by Father energy. Sometimes we just want to surrender, to let go of everything that feels like "me" and to merge with something cosmic or universal. The world is too much with us, and we want to empty out. Or when circumstances bring us to our knees, sometimes there is nothing left to do but drop.

The experience of surrendering to simplicity, of accepting that we are uncomplicated, is blissful! It is a profound release.

Being simple may feel like silence, emptiness, and space. It may feel intimate. It may feel lonely. Many people are afraid of emptiness. When we just let ourselves be, we are letting down the walls of our usual defenses. We let go of effort, the pressure to perform, the ways we control. Our boundaries soften, and the old masks fall away. This different sense of self takes a little getting used to. You may feel undefended, skinless, young, or like your brain has turned to mush. But when you learn to relax into the emptiness, it becomes permission, a palpable spaciousness (ah, space to breathe!) that is deeply restful. Learn to welcome the strange yet familiar quality. Within it is a clue to your serenity.

LISTENING AND WAITING

Simplicity is the art of listening and waiting. Here in the so-called modern world, time and attention are jam-packed with activity. It can take a while in meditation for us to unravel enough to be able to hear. If you wait and listen patiently, eventually your soul will sing.

Over the course of our lifetimes each of us develops ways to fend off the pains and pressures of living. We create a kind of protective shell that helps us get through difficult times. But often this shell persists long after it is needed, and serves only to cut us off from life. The "shell" is actually made of mental, physical, and emotional habits of blocking out experience, and this denial pattern becomes wired into the nervous system. Underneath this armor is our authentic self, the self we are when we truly relax.

Human beings are very inventive when it comes to creating ways to relax. We unwind through sex, sports, movies, TV, books, booze, and drugs—to name a few. The need to let go is so real and so great that some of these methods are used to excess, often damaging our health in the process. Relying only on these outer behaviors prevents the basic inner pattern from ever changing.

Meditation is a way to unravel safely and consciously. The advantage of meditation, especially in the manner we are suggesting, is that the unwinding happens very deep in your nervous system, down at the level where true change occurs.

Letting go of who we think we are is a beautiful thing—it is also awesome and terrifying. Sometimes grief comes up as we let go. You may realize how much and how long you've been holding on. Let the tears flow; your heart is melting and opening to life. Learn to tolerate the process as old patterns are stripped away; watch your beliefs, your fears, and your disappointments twist and turn on the spindle of awareness. Listen and wait, laugh and cry. Eventually you will be knitted together again from a deeper, truer state.

SIMPLE NATURE

In simplicity attention is freed up from all the effort of doing and being somebody. We are more present and available to receive the impressions of the colors, sounds, and movements of life around us. When we are simple, our hearts are more supple, more open to receive, and even small acts of kindness from another can touch us to the core.

The state of simplicity evokes gratitude—for the simple fact of being alive, for the smallest of pleasures that come our way. We feel innocent; we belong. Meditation lets you appreciate the simple sense of being part of nature; your senses are nature recognizing itself. After meditating, sensory experience becomes vivid and the mundane takes on much more immediacy. The touch of light, the taste of water, even walking across the room—all can seem like miracles. The serenity of simplicity explains why, if you could see into the heart and mind of both a monk walking along a forest trail—owning nothing, expecting nothing—and a lonely billionaire in his penthouse, you would pity the billionaire.

Our friend Georgianne, mother of a five-year-old daughter, Serina, points out that a mother is naturally drawn into simplicity meditations when she has small children. A hundred times a day you are forced to surrender, to slow down and pay attention. When you take a child for a walk, you must slow to her pace, stopping to smell a flower or to watch a bug on a leaf. Every two seconds there is something new to observe. A mother must continually let go, not only of rigid scheduling but in the deepest movement of her heart. The maternal bond is a powerful pri-mordial instinct. Each time a mother hands her baby over to the care of another, she aches with concern for the child's safety; it is a visceral tug on the cords of that bond. Every day is a little death and a challenge to live in trust. When the mother learns to accept this process and allows herself to be changed by it, her heart is softened and stretched. This demonstrates again how women's awareness of the preciousness of life leads us into a natural spirituality that does not have to be manufac-tured or enforced.

A kind of translucency comes with simplicity. The veil between inner and outer becomes sheer, and the obstructions that obscure inti-macy with the world fall away. In this permeability, divine light can pen-etrate us—all the way to the bones. Our own inner radiance shines forth, with no effort, grand design, or demonstration. We simply are—a vessel simultaneously empty and full. We accept our nature—foolish and wise, bounded and boundless, ephemeral and everlasting.

CONFESSION

The privacy of meditation lets us face our deepest secrets. As we are infused with love and acceptance, the parts inside that do not know love and acceptance eventually are touched. Remorse for past actions, regret for lost opportunities, or even core shame is brought to our attention to be confessed and healed. You may burn with embarrassment or cry your guts out with grief, but what a great place to be washed and rinsed clean!

In 1990, shortly after moving to Los Angeles, I had a showdown with my own patterns of control. After fourteen years in Santa Fe, I had been eager to dismantle encrusted identities and open myself to new blood, new life, and more circulation. When I first arrived in the City of Angels, I had exclaimed, "Let the Angels of Change have their way with me!" Well, they surely did. In the flux and unpredictability of L.A. life, things weren't working out quite as I'd hoped, and I was riddled with frustration and doubt. But this I knew: when you can't push the river, you might as well be carried downstream. There was naught to do but submit.

In meditation my "false self" was brought out in Technicolor. Mental habits of "performing" and pumping myself up arose and then dissolved as I let them go. An undercover operation was exposed: a shame still merciless even after so damn much work on myself—shame at imagined failure, shame at being seriously flawed, shame that had no description but felt like hell. A friend asked, "What is the image of your shame?" Immediately it was clear: a retarded girl, simpleminded and drooling.

Having made a career out of inner theater, I was intrigued with this new character. As I meditated with this image, it began to instruct me, and my feeling was soon transformed from humiliation to relief. I let my face soften into her face, my eyes and mouth going completely slack. I let my body become flaccid and amorphous like hers, muscles and fat falling from my bones. Even my brain felt limp. If snot sniveled down my chin, so what? If I never accomplished anything ever again, who cared? I groaned and sighed, giggled and cried as my nervous system unwound. My whole being was relaxing and opening, and I was getting rewired.

As luck would have it—or in another instance of the strange conspiracy between the inner and outer worlds—life presented me with a gift. Lorin and I were at a movie matinee not long after we had reunited following a painful separation. When the lights came up, I saw that sitting behind us was an entire row of Down's syndrome children. They were so happy, unself-conscious, and affectionate. They never stopped touching each other, holding hands, and nudging playfully as they lumbered up the aisle. Here was my image of openness to life: simple-minded, openhearted immediacy and joy. I, of course, burst into tears.

I realized that, because I was always trying so hard, the simple state had been my shadow. I had blocked my simplicity because it had seemed defective, but in fact it is the ability to rest and enjoy. This encounter and my simple girl stay forever close inside my heart, and whenever I forget my simple nature, she is there to remind me with her easy smile. Through her (I confess) I have been truly changed.

REST IN THE ELEMENTS

The primary elements of nature provide qualities that you can rest in. In some systems there are three major elements, in others five. We are sticking with the quaternity of earth, air, water, and fire.

Each element provides a particular healing and nourishing tone and has a special texture or movement. While meditating on an element, you can immerse yourself in its atmosphere—being held by it, absorbed in it, fed by it. Let the element simplify you. Its qualities may permeate you so thoroughly that you even seem to become the element itself. It is a joyous relief to surrender the small, separate self and merge with an aspect of the wise, vast body of the natural world.

Earth grounds, contains, and supports. Earth energy is heavy and deep, like a mountain or cave, or slowly shifting, like sand. You may crave this quality when you are overwhelmed, frenetic, or mentally fried. One of my favorite meditations is to imagine that I am surrounded by warm dark earth, completely contained and unable to move, see, hear, or speak. The sense of weight and stillness is profoundly relaxing and soothing. Sound bizarre? Some people literally enact this image by having themselves buried in sand (with a straw to breathe from) for an hour or more until their friends dig them out. Giving in to earth energy does have something to do with trust!

Air, light and unbounded, moves freely. The touch of air can be a sultry caress on the skin like a tropical breeze, or a bracing tonic like a cool, wild wind. You may crave air as leavening if your heart has been burdened or heavy with grief. In meditation you can imagine a strong wind blowing through you and taking away whatever wants to be released, as if you are on a mountaintop, or at the ocean shore. Or you can meditate with the lightness, spaciousness, and freedom of air—a great antidote when responsibilities have crowded out your joy.

Water flows and cleanses, like the pure streaming of a river, waterfall, or fountain. It encompasses and supports with buoyant strength, like a pool, lake, or sea. You may crave water energy if you have been rigidly controlled, pushing too hard, or feeling dry and isolated. To meditate with the flushing movement of water can refresh and revitalize you. Or you can imagine that you have dissolved into a large body of water and let yourself be carried by it, soaking in its nourishment. When you melt into water energy, you come into an easy flow and sense of connectedness, both within yourself and with those around you.

Fire is expansive and energizing. It provides warmth, protection, and light, and it can be delicate (a candle) or exhilarating (a bonfire). To immerse yourself in the meditative fire can be like entering the heart of the sun or a holy flame that burns you clean. Rest in the fire; let it surround and protect you. Be consumed by flame. Let your mind and heart be purified and strengthened in the fire.

Each element has a purity and simplicity that is a gift and inspiration. Each is a world of experience so sacred and holy that an entire religion could be developed around it—and probably has been! Which element holds a special gift for you?

❧ EXPLORATIONS

- When are you at rest within yourself? In what situations can you just let yourself be?
- With what friends or lovers are you comfortable just being yourself?
- Recall how you've felt after a good cry, how rinsed out and refreshed you were. Your heart was tender, and you could smile again, or even laugh. Maybe the world seemed new, or you fell back in love with your friends. Take a minute and write about one of those times.

&2 **WARM-UP: SIMPLE AWARENESS IN THE WORLD**

Experiment with this at home, sitting in a park or at a restaurant, walking through the airport—anywhere you choose. An anonymous setting can give you a sense of freedom, but you can also practice this awareness with people you know.

With your eyes open, simply take in the world. Let your attention play through the variety of sense impressions as if you have never before experienced them, like a curious alien who's just been incarnated in human form. Enjoy the quality of light, the particular colors, and the shapes and movement that you see. Receive any sounds and let them float into your ears like music. Notice any smells that waft in with your breath. Delight in your own body awareness, the sense of yourself immersed in this rich field of life. If other people are present, let them move around you and just observe and feel them. Let yourself be present, feeling no obligation to respond in any way but feeling free to do so if you get the urge. Keep coming back to the pleasure of your simplest state of being.

- Remember your inner wilderness preserve? What natural environment do you love that evokes a restful state?
- Make a list of all the things you are grateful for.

&2 Skill Circle #9:
HOW TO MEDITATE WITH SIMPLICITY

To allow simplicity to emerge:

- Demand nothing of yourself in the name of meditation. Don't put any pressure on yourself to "perform" in meditation.
- Thoughts will come and go. When you become aware of them, gently bring your attention back to your focus (any of the meditations with breath, sound, or sensation).
- Let your thoughts float by, as if they have no weight to them.
- Keep coming back to the simple pleasure of your chosen meditation and let yourself rest inside the atmosphere it creates. Take in every pleasurable detail. In this way you will cultivate that new state of being.

Some days when you sit down in your meditation spot, silence will settle over you. Especially if you've been meditating every day for a while, a tangible, physical presence of peace can show up as soon as you start to settle in, even with your eyes still open. At these times, don't feel that you need to do any technique or even close your eyes. Just sit there and be with the silence. Meet it. This unexpected serenity, a condition of complete simplicity, occurs to meditators at any level—beginner, intermediate, or advanced. There is no need to complicate this state by adding a technique.

> 🎜 **TIP**
>
> Take a nap and then meditate.

Reinvent Your Approach

Resting in simplicity is a way to begin anew in meditation, to unravel old ways of being and find the way to meditate that is congruent with who you are today. We all need to stay current with ourselves and to allow our meditation approach to change as we do.

A meditation technique is intended to lead beyond itself into "doing nothing." It is something very simple and gentle that we do to help us go beyond *doing* into *being*. Usually we can't just sit and do nothing, so techniques are really useful. However, just from habit, we often bring a sense of effort to the meditation technique; our grip is too tight. Underlying this tendency are several factors: our patterns of avoidance and control always try to take hold, and whatever attitude we had when we started doing that technique will persist.

One day in the late 1960s Lorin was meditating, and as usual at the end of a meditation, he sat with his eyes closed for a couple of minutes. This time he noticed that in the transition time after doing the technique he actually went deeper into being. "I saw that I had been making a minuscule amount of effort to stay with technique, and just that hint of doing was keeping me from experiencing being. The total simplicity had eluded me. I didn't even know it was there waiting for me."

Later, as a meditation teacher, he realized that this is a common problem with advanced meditators. They cling too tightly to the technique because they are trying to "do it right." Or an old technique may no longer be needed or may even be causing stagnation. Sometimes they use the technique as a kind of spell to ward off pain or edit out parts of themselves they don't like. But what they end up blocking out is actually their own being, that still small voice within that knows exactly what they need.

Coming back to simplicity gives you the opportunity to let go and reinvent yourself in meditation. Therefore, it's useful to have meditation times when you use no technique at all. Just show up and be available to yourself. Keep coming back. Every now and then practice "doing nothing."

The Do-Nothing Technique

In this exercise, you sit or lie down and simply be with yourself without any agenda. For five or ten minutes give your attention free rein to go anywhere. Accept yourself completely. Nothing has to be other than it is; you do not have to be other than you are right this moment. This helps you get used to the idea that you can rest in simplicity—with no need to make something happen, no need to control.

Practice not manipulating yourself in any way in meditation. It can be a stretch to tolerate your natural and unembellished state. Notice where your mind goes; notice the feelings that come up. Find out what happens when you release control.

🥨 MEDITATIONS

Breath Meditation: No Demands

This can be done sitting comfortably or lying down. If you sit, you could prop lots of cushions around you to feel cozy. If you lie on the floor, let your legs be slightly open, and you may want to put a pillow under your knees to relieve your lower back.

Take time just to settle in and notice your internal climate. Then become aware of your breath, just as it is, without changing it in any way. Be with the rhythm and texture of the breath and rest in that awareness.

After several minutes, become aware of your whole body and begin to imagine that the breath takes on the shape of your form. Each breath flows in and gently and effortlessly fills every nook and cranny, from your toes to the tips of your fingers. As you exhale, relax. Do this for several breaths, then let the attention go and simply feel. Come back every once in a while to take a few conscious breaths that fill your entire form, then let go again and rest.

After ten minutes or so, keeping your eyes closed, bring your attention back to the breath and your body and begin to become aware of the environment around you: the room you're in, the sounds, the touch of the air. Letting your body stay relaxed inside, slowly open your eyes. Take in the quality of the light, colors, and shapes. Simply receive the impressions for several minutes without having to do anything. Continue to make a very gradual transition. Gently wiggle your fingers and toes, stretch a little bit, take a couple of deep breaths. As you emerge and get up to stand and walk, observe how different your body feels.

Gratitude Meditation

Often we are grateful but do not take time to let the feeling wash through and change us. In this meditation, explore your gratitude more deeply. Happy people make a point of thinking about what they are grateful for; they fall in love with the simplest things.

From the items on your gratitude list, take one at a time and ponder it for a minute. Gently turn the image of that item in your mind and see everything about it. Let your body and breath interact with the state the image evokes—the feeling in your heart, the way all of your senses open up, the way your eyes take in the world, how you breathe. How does the gratitude change you?

Continue with two or three other things you are grateful for. Then let the images fade away and be there in the aftereffect of all the sensations and feelings. The power of gratitude may break your heart. You may melt inside; you may feel sorrow from missing what you're grateful for; you may gurgle with joy.

Then let go of all that and sink into the silence. Simply rest in yourself. It is in this afterglow that your nervous system can be reorganized.

❧ SHARE THE WEALTH

To more fully embrace what you are grateful for, meditate on spreading that quality around. You can add the tag line: "May my abundance (joy, prosperity, peace, and so on) serve and inspire others. . . ."

This meditation orients your cells, your whole body, toward what you really cherish. Follow and study the scent of your gratitude. This lets you learn to be in a state of expansion and gratitude for what you've already experienced. It also alerts your body to be open to the gifts that the future will bring.

&* GOING FURTHER

Meditation with Earth, Air, Water, and Fire

What element do you crave? What image comes to mind? You can meditate with the elements through outward or inward attention.

In outward attention you focus on some form of the element and let your senses receive from it. For example, if earth energy calls, you can nestle down on the ground, sit on a rock or the sand, and meditate with the kinesthetic sense of gravity. Explore the feeling of foundation, solidity, and containment. With air, you can lie on your back and gaze at the sky, releasing into the spaciousness as you take in the casual drift of clouds or the infinity of stars at night. With water, you can meditate near a fountain, stream, lake, or ocean and listen to its refreshing sound, watching its movement and the shimmering play of light on its surface. Small portable fountains can be purchased for inside your home to provide the sound and flow of water energy. If you crave the fire element, sit in contemplation of a candle or the fire in your hearth and take in the color and dance of flame. You can also hear its crackle or hiss and feel its radiant warmth.

To meditate inwardly, call up an image of that element, something that seems nourishing or energizing. Contemplate it just as you would if you saw it outwardly. Then imagine that you are merging with the image, placing yourself inside of it. The image may change in some way as you find what satisfies you. As the element envelops you, rest within. Immerse yourself thoroughly in the elemental substance: become earth or fire or air or water.

In either mode, receive the energy from the element you crave. Let it "in-form" you: let your own form take on its qualities. Become one with it completely. To merge with the elements is a powerful and healing meditation. When you are ready to emerge, take time to appreciate the different sense of yourself and your body from this in-forming. As a gentle transition, open and close your eyes a few times, stretch a little bit, and when you come to standing and walking, explore any new awareness.

✥ REFLECTIONS

- As you explore the simplicity meditations, which one is particularly satisfying? Let yourself get used to that satisfaction.
- What body sensations do you notice as you relax and release?
- Does anxiety, worry, or fear come up? What is the taboo you may be breaking? What permission can you give yourself?

✿ SECRET #10
DO NOT FEAR THE DEPTHS

I've had it. Too much, too much world.
Don't want to do anything, don't want to see anyone.
Is something wrong with me? Am I depressed?
Well, no, not really. I just need to let go,
Let down, get down—down to my inner roots.

Let my meditation take me down,
Down beneath the surface chatter,
Under the clatter and clutter of human design.
Ugh, my eyes burn with the excess of light.
My ears ache with the weight of words.
No more to give, to say, to hear . . .
I crave silence. I crave darkness.
I want to dissolve in darkness.
I want to disappear . . .

Turn off all the lights, seal myself in sanctuary,
Give in to the downward pull.
Into the dark body of Earth I descend . . .
Ah, Darkness, immerse me in your silence.
Surround me in your velvet embrace.
With blackness and eternity I merge. I dissolve . . .
All that remains is this breath . . . and this . . .
Take what you will. I offer this to you . . .

Slowly, slowly, the return to life . . .
I am . . . somehow different, somehow re-created

Out of the fertile dark unknown.
I died to my old self, yet I feel more myself than ever—
More . . . authentic, deeper, real. And strangely free.
A hint of possibility, a whisper of something new,
And a subtle, simple, shameless joy.

❧ ❧ ❧

GOING DOWN, MA'AM?

There is an ebb and flow to experience, crests and valleys of emotion and energy level. In the course of even one day a woman can move through any number of these up-and-down cycles. Whether they are emotional reactions to outward circumstances, the fluctuations of hormones, or the simple self-balancing of our bodies and brains, these dips and surges are necessary and natural. Nobody complains about the ups; it's the downs of the cycle we need to learn to accept. Here's the rub: if we do not give in to them, the valleys accumulate and compound into an even deeper plunge. Meditation keeps track of our little daily rhythms and also helps us to comply with the longer, more precipitous descents.

Just to let go after a period of intense work is a "let-down" and can feel like sadness. Maybe you're simply tired and need a rest. Maybe you're a little blue because you woke up with a weird dream or a nagging sense that a personal interaction went sour. Maybe you had a massage that loosened up old feelings that you haven't had a chance to process. Whatever the cause, something is coming up and you're being pulled down.

The better part of valor is to stop, drop inward and face yourself, face reality, and be changed by the experience. It's a mini-meltdown of how we hold ourselves together—a little death and surrender of identity through which we are reorganized and revived. This downward movement is part of the deep psychological ecology of the feminine. Consciousness is being called under the surface to feed, weed, and re-seed the inner world. Going down reflects an innate wisdom that we can—and must—remember to trust.

This trust, however, flies in the face of our collective social values. We rejoice in the periods of enthusiasm, uplift, and outward productivity; these values are enshrined by our culture. But the valleys—the organic movements downward and inward—are shrouded in judgment and fear. We meet them with anxiety and a perverse certainty that something is terribly wrong. In most cases, nothing could be further from the truth.

Because of this gross misunderstanding, the subtle tug inward is often dismissed—or worse, pathologized. The inner call goes unanswered and unfulfilled; its cries become louder and more insistent, its symptoms more intense. Not knowing that this downward pull is healthy and natural, and not being educated in how to honor this state, women flock to external authorities to make the feeling go away. Pharmacologists are kept busy; the marketing of antidepressants is now a cornerstone of our corporate economy. Sometimes medical intervention is appropriate, but too often it is used to mask the deeper need. The call inward and downward is genuine and entirely normal. We all need to let go, over and over again.

THE MOVEMENT OF SOUL

There are times in a woman's life when the call downward is a transformative journey, a summons to the depths of the soul.

People tend to think of spirituality as rising upward into the sky. In the traditional (male) teachings, enlightenment is often described as a flight from the lower centers in the body, the instinctive and sexual places, to the upper centers in the head and then out. By contrast, a woman's spiritual quest at some point leads to a soulful sinking down into herself. Everyone fears this descent, this sinking down. Yet sinking down connects us with the earth, with our personal ground, with our foundation. There is a secret in "endarkenment."

The realm of the soul is not light and airy, but more like mud: messy, wet, and fertile. Soul processes go on down there with the moss and worms, down there with the decaying leaves, down there where death turns into life. Deepening into soul requires the courage to go underground, to stretch our roots into the dark, to writhe and curl and meander through rich, moist soil. In this darkness we find wisdom, not through the glaring beam of will, but by following a wild, blind yet unfailing instinct that senses the essence in things, that finds nourishment to suck back into growth.

Rare is the man who can take it. That's why male spirituality is so often about getting out of the mess, about transcending the passions and bloody processes of life. Who can blame them, really? It takes a woman's body and strength of spirit for this journey.

At some time in your unfolding, you will make this journey.

THE MYSTERY OF DESCENT

In classical mythologies, from the Sumerian to the Greek, female initiations involve a descent into the underworld with a return to normal life after a profound transformation. While our heroine is in the underworld, all hell breaks loose. In Sumerian myth, Innanna, Queen of Heaven, hears the mourning cries of her dark sister, Ereskigal, the goddess of the underworld. When she descends to meet her, she is stripped, flayed, and hung by Ereskigal on a bloody hook to rot. When she is finally returned to the surface, Innanna is a little darker, deeper, and wiser. When the Greek goddess Persephone is abducted by Hades, she disappears from life. In her distress, Persephone's mother, Demeter, goddess of grain and growth, grieves inconsolably, neglects her fields, and lets them die. Persephone resurfaces but is sentenced to return to Hades six months of every year. In shamanistic imagery, healing requires a journey into the death realm to retrieve the part of the soul that is lost, and without which one cannot be truly alive. Only after this descent and soul retrieval can transformation and resurrection take place.

Modern-day women who have been exploring meditation say that there are phases of the journey that feel just like death and dismemberment. This is the death of the false self, constructed of the illusions that are unique for each woman: the dutiful daughter, the ingenue, the sex kitten, the control freak, the mistrustful misanthrope, the long-suffering martyr, the all-powerful queen. Some outmoded image has got to go. We know it, but it's hard to let it die. The more we try to pump up our usual reality, the more dissatisfying it becomes; something just does not feel right. The fields are fallow and dry because life force is drawing us down to our roots. Eventually we descend.

The pull downward may feel like depression or as though the bottom is dropping out of your psyche. When you feel that downward pull, however, know that soul is calling. Cooperate with it. Your meditation practice is the perfect place to allow the descent to fulfill itself.

SOLITUDE, SORROW, AND THE SACRED WELL

The downward-moving emotions, such as regret, grief, and loneliness, lead you into your depths. Everyone experiences these at times during meditation, and they are not to be resisted. If you have undergone the loss of a loved one, a way of life, a self-image, or a dream, there may be grief in your heart. Enter the grief and let it release its healing gift.

When we are in solitude or in sorrow, we are sitting by the sacred well of life. Although we may be crying, we will emerge renewed. Though we fear we could cry forever, the more we yield to this process, the more quickly it can resolve itself. Many meditators say there are times when they die and are reborn in a heartbeat because they have learned to surrender.

In opening to our own suffering, we share in the poignancy of the human condition. We become aware of others who suffer, tuning in to the morphogenetic field of humanity. Linking to the rest of humanity through our shared suffering can be a conscious prayer and transformation. In meditation we can open our hearts to breathe in the suffering of the world and to breathe out with compassion and healing for the self and others.

Grief and love are intertwined. If you love, you risk inevitable loss—and choose to love regardless. We lose each other one way or another, through separation or death. To bear this grief is to live with an open heart.

DEPRESSION

When we hear the word *depression,* we all have a sense of its meaning, but this oft-used term hints at many different conditions. True depression is a long descent, painful and complex. Aside from brain chemistry and hormones, what is going on? Let's explore some of the facets of depression to see whether we can get inside it and find the secret buried within the darkness.

If we've been abducted into the underworld, we may feel betrayed by life and, like Innanna, as though we've been stripped bare, our skin flayed, and our limbs ripped off and hung on hooks deep inside a cave. We are sure we will never emerge; eternity has us in its grip. How will we ever see the light of day? What must we learn to be resurrected and transformed?

Most women carry more stress than they realize. Sustained stress exhausts the body's energy supply. Depression naturally follows as the body attempts to shut down nonessential functions to recharge. In depression you don't want to do anything, you don't want to go outside, you don't want to see anybody. Your energy is sapped, and you feel powerless to change. You just want to sit in the dark, symbolically or literally. If you're depressed, you probably have a profound need to rest.

Some women have discovered that depression serves another important function: giving them privacy. Especially if your family system was invasive or denied the depths of feeling, depression creates an inner retreat. It may be your only way to justify your need for solitude and sit at the sacred well of your own being.

On the other hand, isolation and lack of intimacy can be heart-rending factors in depression. The physical and psychological need for touch is little recognized. One friend observed: "Sometimes what is going on is that the woman's outer life has to change, not just her inner, but that seems overwhelming or impossible. The cause of her depression is a very real, very profound dissatisfaction. She is lonely, she needs to move away, find community; she needs a relationship, someone to love and to hold."

The root of depression may be a craving for simplicity. We may be so overwhelmed that we just want to give up. Depression, especially during times of transition such as midlife, often involves a desire to die to the old self. Thoughts of suicide, the ultimate act of giving up, may arise, but they are not to be taken literally. Almost all women who have such thoughts never act on them. But they are urgent clues that some deep surrender must take place. The depths of your being are calling. Do not resist the call.

The words themselves hold within them the release: *give up, give in, give over, give away*. We need to unburden ourselves from old ways of being and doing that are no longer appropriate. We must give in to the desire to simplify our lives. This can feel like a sacrifice, and it is. It can feel like a death, and it is. Place those old parts of yourself on your inner altar; let them be sacrificed so that new life can flow.

Angelique resides in New Mexico and by nature is deeply spiritual. She is an artist who specializes in "life as art." She curates, creates performances and ritual-pilgrimages for the earth, and practices healing breath-work. At age fifty-six, Angelique found herself suddenly and profoundly depressed. Despite the urging of her concerned therapist friends, she decided not to take medication and intuited her own path instead.

As Angelique courageously explored the lifeless state, she came to accept the descent and allowed herself to be dismantled and transformed. To come to terms with her own death, she began to live as if she had only a year to live, a practice of conscious living and dying articulated by Stephen Levine. Angelique cooperated with the metamorphosis, facing her grief and fear as a new strength grew within. Gradually she released all that no longer had meaning for her. Now, a year later, she has emerged simplified and renewed. She feels more alive than ever, clarified, and truly emancipated. "Now that it is behind me, I see that a two-year descent was necessary for my psyche to break through the old doors of limitation. I may be a little more tender . . . but I welcome this tenderness—the emerging cocoon for the heart I always knew was my path. This return is about closure and resolution. . . . Comfort at last. At the same time, it is a place of emergence where

❧ RACHEL'S STORY: ENTERING THE UNKNOWN

When we are in the underworld, the membrane between the inner and outer worlds is very sheer, and we become sensitive to the mystery of the unknown.

Rachel, an attractive woman in her early fifties, had been plagued by depression for years. She had long been fighting off a call to descend. Living in Paris and working in finance, Rachel found that when her marriage fell apart, so did her identity. Returning to the United States, she writes, was "an excruciating experience of being lost and alone, not knowing what I was doing or what I was supposed to be doing.

"Then I began having dreams—powerful dreams teaching me things I didn't know in waking life. 'Listen to your true self,' dream after dream was saying. But the only inner voice I knew when awake was harsh, judgmental, and critical, the one that had been screaming and cajoling in my head for most of my life. This voice told me to fear my inner depths, dismissed my dreams as brain irregularities, and scorned my insights as signs of madness. This voice wanted to drug me out of the curse of myself through every prescribed antidepressant and anti-anxiety medicine that came on the market. None of them worked.

"I knew I had to discover a voice long forgotten, lost, and shamed into hiding. I didn't even know what I was searching for. I just knew that I had to dig, and dig deep—a kind of excavation of my soul. Though my life as I'd known it was disintegrating, I kept trying to regroup. A new project. New relationship. New therapy. New home. But depression and despair, hopelessness and loss of heart, always drew me back to the dig.

"In meditation with Camille I learned to explore this place without trying to understand or change it. I was learning to see without shaming myself, which always leads to depression. During the long process, the enormous inner struggles and upheavals, it often felt as if I were digging my own grave. As I sank deeper into the sea of not knowing, the remaining structures of my life—those that defined me as daughter, lover, friend, artist, non-artist, depressed

I have the choice and the impetus to create my life anew—what a great blessing."

Living with awareness of our mortality is a powerful ongoing meditation. In many traditions preparation for death is the foundation of spiritual practice. We would caution, however, that what may well be calling is life itself. There is a danger in being too spiritual: premature dissolving of the self. For many women, succumbing and dying back is too easy when surrender to their own creativity is the real need. Living fully can be far more spiritual, more courageous and challenging. The key is to live *your* life, not someone else's idea of how you should be.

You can create rituals for the descent. Simple acts of letting go may suffice: give away old possessions that feel too much, too heavy; responsibility that feels too much, too heavy; activities that feel too much, too heavy. Let the ritual of releasing them lighten your heart.

---

patient, wounded healer, student, teacher, feminist, mystic, you name it—dissolved. I became mute—there was nothing to say about the experience. Everything was muted and shadowy.

"Sometimes I would curl up under a blanket in a fetal position, and eventually I heard something small, barely a whisper. A still small voice, long ago buried and forgotten, was calling me from the very depths of my being, the feminine wisdom, the sustained and generative knowing of myself as a woman. Slowly, from a place deep within myself, energy began to move through my arms and hands in spontaneous gestures. The inner movement seemed to shape my body into archetypal poses—Balinese dancer, an ancient priestess, feline prowling. Something elemental was beginning to move me—something primordial, bestial. Words were annoyances, mere sounds that made no sense in my animal world and got in the way of listening. I was after something deeper, something beneath words. Some deep force of my being was rebuilding me. Though it felt formless, it wasn't chaotic. It just *was*.

"Over time I was moved out of the experience of pure being, but not back into doing. Instead, the tension between being and doing created a loom on which *becoming* wove itself into new shapes and patterns. It was as if I had dissolved into a place of forming, a paradox: an empty place, filled with the pulse of life, a place of becoming, the furnace of creation. I learned to identify with this process of creation and stopped trying to revive my old identities. 'Not knowing' no longer frightened me into submission, depression, and fear—it no longer elicited anxiety. I was too absorbed in the process of creation itself. I was alive and curious.

"The experience of being moved from the inside out, shaped and re-formed from deep within myself, also seemed to open me up, to create more space within which things could happen—both on the inside and in the world around me. My mind and heart are being urged open, and as a result, something has emerged that's able to synthesize what is important to me in the moment. I can now tolerate the ambiguity and trust the mystery of the process of which I've become an integral part."

Down and Out

When a person feels powerless to answer her inner call and is trapped in the circumstances of her life, the body and psyche resort to dramatic, metaphoric measures. If energy cannot be expressed or fulfilled, madness, illness, and even death can provide a way out. Classical psychology sees a link between depression and suppressed anger; when rage can't be outwardly expressed, the anger turns in toward the self. The madwoman is an archetype of this conundrum. Her madness is a theatrical demonstration of qualities that scream to be acknowledged, a one-woman show of what must be accepted by her family or society—and most important, by herself.

Illness can be another symbolic expression of tension, a psychological message not only for the individual but for the whole system she lives in. Our bodies and psyches do not exist in isolation; they are always part of the larger social body, the body politic. A new field of study, "metaphoric illness," examines symptoms as a poetic embodiment of a cultural malaise that has not yet found other means with which to express itself. Chronic fatigue, for example, could be a collective body response to speeded-up modern society, an attempt to bring the dangers of its manic pace to shared consciousness so that we might all get the point and change.

Death, of course, is the final way out, and sometimes it can seem like the only exit from intolerable psychic pain. Suicide expresses not just hopeless surrender but the will to be free. Paradoxically, so obviously self-destructive a choice is also an unconscious act of power. Sometimes suicide is a succinct display of unspoken anger or resentment, reflecting a hidden self-assertion. If you know someone in the grip of this conundrum, take the situation seriously and urge her to get professional help. With the solid support of a health-care professional, she can get in contact with the deeper feelings within the suicidal impulse. She can integrate the secret power, harness the desire to be free, and bring that freedom into life.

At the junction between life and death we are in the vortex where creation and destruction intertwine, in the realm of the goddess whom the Hindus call Kali. Creation cannot happen without destruction. Brought to consciousness, death is the quintessential teacher. Life-threatening illnesses or traumas are wake-up calls, one way or the other.

It is extremely potent to ask, "If I were to die now and be reincarnated, what quality of life would I create?"

❧ EXPLORATIONS

- How tired are you? Many people operate on a sleep deficit. Working mothers may have a sleep debt of twenty hours or more. Take naps. Go to bed early. Rest whenever you can.
- Are you in a transitional period? What new life are you moving into? What is it you must let go of? What is it you must accept?
- What losses and disappointments have you suffered? Consider writing about those events in your journal and perhaps sharing them with a friend. Let the flow of words help release the pain in your heart.
- A joke is circulating on the Internet: "Depression is merely anger without enthusiasm." Is there something you are secretly angry about? Write your true feelings in your journal. Endorse your anger enthusiastically and let its energy move out onto your page.
- What dream images haunt you? What message do they hold?

❧ SKILL CIRCLE #10:
HOW TO CREATE RITUAL

Rituals are symbolic actions that honor and empower times of transition. They are a conscious yes to transformation, a signal to yourself and the powers-that-be that you are willing to change. Rituals are acts that integrate body and soul, so some physical expression is important.

- What is the symbolic meaning of your time of transition? What sort of ritual would be appropriate for marking it?
- Certain actions can satisfy the inner call. For instance, write your own prayer or poem, then speak it out loud. Light a special candle and let the flame embody your desire. Give away something that used to be precious to you but no longer fits who you are. Clean

❧ WARM-UP: DARK EYES

- It is very healing and nourishing for the eyes to be in total darkness, taking a break from the business of seeing. From time to time place your hands over your eyes to seal out the light. Press the base of the palms very gently into your eyelids. Relax your eyes and let them absorb the soothing blackness and the energy from your hands.

out your closets. Bury or burn something. Drip your menstrual blood into the earth. Howl or wail at the moon. Go barefoot in the mud. Plant a garden. Buy yourself flowers. Buy new shoes for your new feet.

• Create a special altar. Think of it as a mirror of your soul. You can keep it really simple, with one object or two, or let it be elaborate and extravagant. Draw upon the bounty of nature, in all four elements: earth, air, water, and fire. Bring in twigs, leaves and rocks, a wooden dish of dirt. Find beautiful feathers; fill a bowl or shell with water; burn at least one candle. Splurge on a new vase. What flowers would be perfect for this time? Add sculptures of goddesses, mirrors, crystals, or sacred talismans. Anything and everything can become meaningful. If you are a writer, place a pen and paper on your altar, or your favorite book. Let this creation evolve over time with the changes of your inner world.

• As if you are going to die within a year, write letters to people you care about, or with whom you feel unresolved. Finish business. Let go of the old. Clean the slate.

• Your meditation time is ritual space. It provides a sacred circle for your descent. Do the meditations here and also those from Secret #7 ("Ride Your Rhythms"). As the Sufis say, "Die before you die." Practice dying in meditation, and reincarnate into your life with new values.

• Wear a ritual garment to meditate. Use a special dress, robe, or shawl to wrap yourself up in the feeling you crave. A fur coat, leather jacket, or skimpy negligee may be just the thing to do the trick.

• Sometimes what is called for is community to relieve your sense of isolation. Participate in a class or group, or enter the sacred circle of therapy if the pain is too great to bear on your own.

• Gather friends for a meditation or ritual circle. Honor the tone you long for. It can be a silent communion, a gentle verbal sharing, or a wild and raucous liberation, busting through old taboos. Draw or paint, sculpt figures in clay. Create an altar together. Get naked outdoors in the sun or under the moon. Build a bonfire or plunge into a lake. Paint your faces and dance, drum, or sing. Shake, rattle, and roll your way into new territories of expression.

❧ MEDITATIONS

The Breath Beyond

This breath releases and dissolves old structures. Called the "Lunar Breath" in Continuum, it is similar to the Ujayi breath in yoga. Combine this with any of the other descent meditations, or use it anytime you want to slow down and let go.

Do this sitting or lying on the floor with pillows under your knees to relieve your lower back. Make sure you are warm and comfortable so that you can deeply relax.

After you get settled, bring your attention to your breath and simply ride its movement for several minutes. Then become more aware of the emptying flow of the exhalation. Begin to elongate the exhalation and, with your mouth closed, make a quiet whispering sound inside your throat. Constrict slightly at the back of your throat, and you will feel the passage of air narrowing to create the sound. Exhale with this sound as slowly as possible. Empty the breath out completely, and wait.

The inhalation will come without any effort on your part. When it does, let it fill you gently. Then exhale again with the whispering breath. With each exhalation, imagine that your usual sense of self dissolves with the out-breath, as though diffused like a fragrance into space. This diffuse awareness is as gentle as moonlight, cooling and spacious rather than solar and direct. Drift beyond the veil of appearances into this cool dark expanse. Release yourself like a cloud into the open night sky.

Belly to the Ground

This simple meditation is very soothing and regenerative and wonderful to do outside on the grass when weather permits. Indoors, choose a soft surface—carpet or several blankets on the floor.

Lie belly down on the ground. Find the most comfortable position for your body. Spread your legs out and nuzzle your pubic bone, belly flesh, and breasts into the ground. Make a pillow with your hands and turn your head to rest on them. (Periodically turn your head to the other side to relieve neck strain.)

As you breathe, let your weight begin to drop and relax the whole front of your body into contact with the ground. With each exhalation, sink down and relax a little more. Notice the swelling movement of the breath inside your skin as it presses gently into the skin of the earth. The body of the planet curves broadly beneath you, and as your body melts into that contact, imagine that you are spreading out and around that huge round expanse. Let the earth breathe into you.

Now as you exhale, open your mouth and let some sound flow down into the ground—a sigh, or groan, or whisper. Let the earth hear you; tell her anything with your sound. Is there something you want to let go of? Send it out with your breath; feel how the old energy flows down and right out of your body. With every exhalation, release yourself more completely.

As you inhale, you receive from the earth's energy; as you exhale, you let go. Honor the tenderness and openness of your underbelly, and with each breath, deepen into soft communion with the earth.

There will be times when you simply rest and the breath moves without your conscious attention. Let that happen and just be. Whenever you feel replete, very gently and gradually begin to stir and nuzzle back into your life.

❧ GOING FURTHER

Down to the Bone Meditation

Your bones are the very core of your structure. They compose the scaffolding for your muscles, skin, and organs, a latticework of support. Everyone has an image of the skeleton; we've seen enough of them at Halloween. But you may be unaware that living bone is not brittle and desiccated, but resilient, moist, and continually regenerating. The minerals in your bones were created from the explosive death of supernovae; imagine that starlight still permeates your cells.

The substance of bone is enduring; even after death and the ravages of time, the bones remain. The Tibetan tradition includes many meditations on the decomposition of the flesh that are intended to help the meditator disidentify from life in the body, for instance, by meditating at graveyards or drinking from human skulls. Here we are concentrating on the profound release of getting down to the bones, paring down to the essence and innermost structure of your being—that which remains when all else falls away.

Doing this meditation in complete darkness is wonderful. Seal your room from any light or cover your eyes with a blindfold, eye pillow, or cloth. Subtle music, very soft, spacious, and unimposing, can help you let go (see the recommendations at the end of the book). Lie on your back to begin. If you like, place a bolster under your knees and a small pillow under your head if your neck is tight. Make sure the room is warm or cover yourself with a blanket so that you can deeply let go. You can do all these steps, or just some of them.

Step 1 Nestle the back of your waist and hips into the ground; nuzzle the back of your chest and shoulders into the floor. Roll your head gently side to side and release the weight of your head. Scan the entire back surface of your body to spread it open into contact with the ground. Give over your weight, soften the back of your throat and the inside of your mouth, let your chin drop and your teeth separate slightly. Release and soften the back of your heart.

Now bring your attention to your breath and begin to focus on the exhalation. Exhale very slowly through your nose or mouth and hear the sound of your breath. With each breath, drop your weight down through your back a little more. Feel your muscles drip from your bones into the floor. Release your bones; let them fall back into the bones of the earth. Imagine your flesh dissolving away so that only the bones remain. Give yourself an eternity to let go.

Step 2 Engage your inner vision to imagine the structure of your bones. See them as if through an X-ray, highlighted against the darkness. Dwell with that perception for several minutes.

Step 3 Begin to create a subtle vibration in your bones through vocal sound. Explore the buzzing consonants such as *vvvv* or *gggg* (as in "Gigi") or *zzzz,* or any combination of them. Feel and imagine the vibration penetrating into your bones. After stimulating them with the sound for a minute or two, relax again and notice the aftereffect.

Step 4 Very gently come to a sitting position. Let your skeleton move to stack itself up, and let your flesh simply drape from this inner foundation. Continue to meditate on this simplified and essential state. The bones are at your core, hidden from public view; they are a private and secret strength. Envision their luminosity from your skull all the way to your feet.

Very slowly begin to return. Open your eyes to the dark and absorb the impressions. As you prepare to move again, feel your bones as support, fed by the support of the bones of the earth. Know how enduring and virtually indestructible this inner structure is—beyond superficial reality, beyond time, beyond death.

Descent to the Goddess Meditation

Sometimes you are called to the underworld—not just once but at many junctures in your life. As an initiate into the mysteries, you can consciously choose to descend to the realm of the dark feminine. This meditation employs your imaginal ability, which leads you out of the tyranny of the literal and down to the poetic truth of soul.

You can sit upright, lie belly down, or lie on your back. Take plenty of time to drop in and become present to yourself. As you relax, your breath will gradually lengthen and slow. When it does, invoke the power of your imagination. Ask it to reveal through this journey exactly what you must know at this time. Then begin your descent. Let any image come as you sink down beneath the surface of the earth. Where are you taken—into a cave, under the water, to the fiery core?

As you arrive, look around and take in the environment. Be surprised by whatever images come. Every detail is important information. You may have to wait until summoned, or you may be greeted immediately by the figure or voice of an underworld goddess, or by a messenger who will take you to her.

When the dark goddess comes, take in everything about her presence. Listen intently; watch carefully. In your imaginal body, bow, gesture, or speak to her. Show her what is in your heart. She may respond in words, sing, dance, touch you, or give you an object. What she says or does may shock you; it may make sense immediately, or it may take some contemplation. Receive whatever teaching she offers, and then, when the time is right, return to the surface.

As you slowly make your way back to ordinary consciousness, sit for several minutes to absorb what transpired. Then write or draw the impressions of what you saw, heard, and felt. When you make a soul journey of this kind, be sure to honor the experience as the revelation that it is. Make a conscious decision to remember and value the images that come and return to them in your meditations from time to time.

Egyptian Pose

In Egyptian initiations, priestesses would lie in a sarcophagus and consciously enter the death realm, returning with visions and dreams. This meditation is a voluntary mini-death and reincarnation. You let go completely and return renewed. This is a good one to do when you feel depressed, disoriented, dreamy, or depleted—and when you suspect that spirit calls.

You can combine this with the "Breath Beyond." If you like, set a timer or use subtle music to keep track of the duration (a half-hour is good). You can also fall asleep in this pose at night and slide right into your dreams.

Cover your eyes and cross your arms over your breasts with one hand on each shoulder (like a mummy). Imagine yourself at the inner depths of an ancient pyramid.

Begin by scanning your body from the feet up, relaxing and releasing each part: the soles, ankles, and toes, your calves, shins, and knees, your thighs and hips, your belly and ribs, your chest and shoulders, your neck, head, and arms. Soften through your scalp and between your brows. Relax your mouth and cheeks. Bring your attention to the area behind your eyes and rest it there lightly for a minute or so.

Now let your mind drift up and away, as if you are looking back at your body from above. Continue to drift away—just let your mind go. There's no need to keep track of anything, so set your consciousness loose.

When you wake up, or at the end of the half-hour, take a generous amount of time to reorient. Slowly come back to consciousness. If images drift back with you, take additional time to reflect upon them.

Imagine that you are reincarnating into a new life. Consider this moment a *tabula rasa,* a clean slate from which you are being re-created, like a work of art. What values now serve as your foundation? What has fallen away and no longer has meaning for you? What texture of life do you want to live and move in? What perceptions, curiosities, desires, or aspirations guide you? What new freedom can you endorse?

Write in your journal as you muse on these questions.

&s REFLECTIONS

- What have you discovered about yourself? What is your relationship to the downward-moving emotions?
- As you let go through these meditations, do you notice any release in your body? Do you feel more grounded, relaxed, closer to the earth?
- What old values are falling away?
- What new values are emerging? How can you acknowledge and express them?

❧ SECRET #11
LOVE YOUR BODY

My left breast is aching.
I sit and breathe and feel, and finally ask:
Why do you hurt? What is it that you need?

Impressions swirl through my awareness, then it is clear:
"You have forgotten me. I am lonely and cold.
I need warmth, and touch."
It is a small plaintive voice, like a furry animal or child.
I say, I hear you, I will give you my touch and warmth.
Please tell me what you want me to know.
I cup my right hand under my breast, my left above.
Immediately the heat of contact floods through my palms
And into the soft tissue with a sigh:
"Too hard, it is too hard. You're always gone.
You push and strive and pull away. I want to be soft.
I don't want to be a warrior's shield.
I want to be held. I want to feel the flow from our heart.
It is right here underneath me, pulsing with warmth and life.
Hold me close so I can let go."

The breast rises and falls, cradled like a baby in my arms.
Longing and grief rise and fall as well
As the breath and warmth weave us together again.
I tell her, I will not forget. I will listen. I will be here with you
Tomorrow and tomorrow—this I vow.
My chest relaxes, my back opens
In the gentle curve of the embrace,
And I begin to feel a presence behind me.

Warmth spreads around my shoulders, behind my heart,
Like wide unfurling wings.
Invisible arms curl around me with soft enfolding flesh.
I am being held; we are being held—
By something ancient, something wise. And I remember:
She is here. She is always here.
We are nestled in the arms of love.

⚃ ⚃ ⚃

BODY SOVEREIGNTY

Loving our own bodies is a challenge for many women. We are so conditioned, nearly hypnotized, to hate our flesh. When our minds are full of imposed ideals, we are in the realm of cultural conditioning. In meditation you enter into the world of sensations beyond the external images, a place where you discover your real body.

Meditation is coming home to yourself. It is recognizing and breathing in your own atmosphere. Dive into meditation to touch your essence, then bring that realization to every part of your body. Use meditation to go beyond the cultural image of a woman's body, and then reperceive your form with wonder and joy.

We are more likely to be able to love our bodies when we are deeply relaxed: just upon waking, if we do not have to get up right away; during a massage; after lovemaking; in the bath. If meditation is equally relaxing, it offers a woman the opportunity to bask in her own love and in the pleasure of simply existing.

Your body is your own. This may seem obvious. But to inhabit your physical self fully, with no apology, is a true act of power. This sovereignty over your body may need to be cultivated. Most of us have been colonized; other people's ideas, desires, and expectations have taken hold in our flesh. It takes some time and effort to reclaim our own terrain. In far too many cases our bodies have been subjected to physical, sexual, or emotional abuse. Sometimes we've abused or neglected ourselves.

Become virgin again. The original meaning of *virgin* referred not to sex but to sovereignty: "She who is unto herself, owned by no one."

Own yourself. Say no when you need to. Only then can you say yes to the ravishment of love.

Through these body meditations you can reestablish your home in yourself. It is a cumulative process that requires compassion, consistency, and commitment. Each time you enter, consciously and tenderly, something within will grow strong and clear. Slowly you will build a new foundation. Every cell will become infused with new consciousness, and the substance of love will become a living reality.

A House United

When, in 1982, I heard of Marion Woodman's book *Addiction to Perfection,* I knew I had to read it; the title says it all. I mention this now to remind you that no matter how painful it has been, your relationship to your body can be redeemed.

Incredible suffering is incurred from the war on the body. The old ideals treat the body—and the self—as an object to be manipulated, berated, and whipped into shape. Shame on you if you fail to live up to perfection—scorn and banishment upon you! If you would just be more disciplined, you could win this battle. This military approach only puts us at war with ourselves—creating a house divided against itself. Military discipline is doomed to failure because what is needed, desperately, is acceptance.

It is continually shocking how painful this area is for most women, even when they see through the fallacious and deadly beliefs. Women often say there is no way they can accept their body as it is, and yet their attempts to alter their form backfire. They are paralyzed, because a wiser but unconscious part of them knows they are in the grip of an internalized, arrogant patriarch and refuses to comply with his demands. Fortitude and a great deal of support are needed to confront that despotic voice and to counter the lies with body wisdom. Only the loving consciousness of the deep feminine is strong enough to break the trance.

Ideals of body image are generic, based in a numbing sense of conformity. These collective images are poisonously laced with a hatred of individuality. This inevitably presents a catch-22: you want to be attractive, and what is attractive is an abstract generic picture. How can you possibly accept your own form and see the beauty in your uniqueness? Impossible! No, not impossible. There are many women who have emancipated themselves and lustily embrace their bodies, no matter what their shape or size. They radiate joy, humor, and gusto—a magnetic power and beauty obvious to all.

If you have the good fortune to be from a family, ethnicity, or culture that accepts and revels in the flesh (and we know there are some of you out there), celebrate wildly, and the rest of us will celebrate on your behalf! We need as many models of healthy embodiment as we can get.

If you are one of the many women who suffer with the image of their body, be patient with yourself. The journey back into your body may bring up anxiety, sorrow, rage, or fear. Sometimes these emotions are the very energy that is being held in, and they literally must move out of your flesh. Expressive movement is one of the best ways for those emotions to be released. Find situations where you feel safe to let them go. The psychic energy behind them will then be liberated to circulate through your whole body as nourishment and vitality.

The Secret of Weight

Ideals of body weight are relative. In many other cultures—Native American, Hawaiian, and Inuit, for example—weight signifies wealth and power, and the more the better! The only problem is that carrying too many extra pounds is not healthy. In our culture heaviness often masks a deep need or desire that isn't getting fulfilled. As a symptom, weight is a symbol or message from your body of an inner craving. Contemplate the literal meaning of weight to find the metaphoric truth inside.

From nature's point of view, fat is fuel. Carrying extra weight is like having your own energy storage, just in case of famine. The big women I know definitely have a lot of psychic energy, a lot of passion and power, though they often have trouble claiming it. Their passions are so strong that they don't know what to do with them. They stuff down their emotions, or numb them out with too much food, or act them out in violent ways. My mother was such a woman; it killed her. I have had to confront her patterns in myself. Learning to dance with volatile energy was one of the main keys to transforming them.

Accept your bigness. Go ahead and be energetically huge; take up lots of physical and psychic space! Meditate on expanding your field: be as broad as a mountain, as vast as the sky. Then your physical body may not have to hold bigness for you unconsciously.

&5 HEALING AND HOOKY

Anne and her husband started a private elementary school in Santa Fe, New Mexico, and have run it for twenty years. The school is highly successful and one of the most respected in the area. She is also a practitioner of *jin shin jyutsu*, and offers this healing advice:

"I like to lie down totally flat and meditate—no pillow. I use a little pillow over my eyes, with lavender. I like to use a mantra while lying down. I go to a totally other place, and then I come back and feel much better.

"All day you get calls—big calls and little calls—to pay attention. When there is something in your body that is really out of balance, those little signals become stronger, and they become more important in informing you what to do. They are always there, but we usually do not pay attention to them. If you want to heal, then you want to make it your business to pay attention.

"You must at times completely let go of outside stimuli and give over to whatever your inner state needs to be. Meditating is the most fun. You let go of the outside stuff and you let the inside come into its own rhythm. There are times you have to go through the residue of depression and anger. Eventually, you get to where you are playing hooky from the world. You feel naughty, because you are having so much fun. Hold on to the hooky feeling. Then afterward when you come out the other side, you feel better. The whole experience is pleasant, even though there are moments that feel dicey.

"If you make a deal with yourself to take this time, and then you don't do it, you create a lack of trust in yourself."

In addition to power and passion, being big and "carrying weight" give a sense of grounding, earthiness, substance, depth, and *gravitas*. Lots of flesh can provide both a feeling of abundance, luxury, softness, and protection, on the one hand, and a painful loneliness or isolation and longing for connection, on the other. These are all *instinctive* needs represented by your flesh: the need for nurturance and love, for rest, nesting, shelter, and communication. Most healers agree that weight is a symptom of stress. Excess weight provides a kind of protective insulation from boundary violations and the other slings and arrows of life. If you struggle with your weight, identify what is stressing you and find new ways to care for yourself. Too much weight is literally a burden on the heart. What heaviness are you carrying, and how might you lighten the load? The deep message may be to learn to receive.

Any dilemma is a dance of opposites, and weight is a dynamic between big and small. So accept your smallness, too. Be vulnerable, innocent and needy; rest in being small. Curl up inside your nest, and give your body what it requires.

Discover the secret within weight, whatever that is for you. Appreciate how devotedly your body has been embodying that message, waiting for you to claim it consciously. If you can accept this, love can flow through your flesh. The war will be over, and the weight will know it is now free to go. It may simply melt away in relief.

Meditate on the metaphor that your body is holding for you. Bask in the quality you crave and learn to satisfy it directly. Find the true nourishment and really take it in. In daily life feed yourself well and take time to enjoy each bite thoroughly. Be soft and tender with yourself. Express your feelings and rally support to make changes in your life where you can. Lay down your burden and get to know the lightness in your heart.

WHERE YOU ARE RIGHT NOW

Watch out for the well-meaning but cryptically perfectionist thought-forms within some New Age healing systems. Many books have become best-sellers by implying that if you only have the right thoughts you will have perfect health and never age. Therefore, if you do find yourself with symptoms of some sort, you obviously have a bad attitude and bad karma and are wearing that scarlet letter in your body for all to see.

Last night I was speaking with my friend Karina. A statuesque woman in her early fifties, she has been a dedicated disciple of a spiritual path for eighteen years. About fifteen years ago Karina was diagnosed with multiple sclerosis. She approaches her condition with philosophical insight, using it as a teaching to accept limitation, to slow down, and to open to the grace within the present moment. Even when giving herself the difficult and painful injections of an ADA-approved drug, she considers it a daily *puja,* or devotional ritual—chanting and blessing the syringes and bottles as if they were the finest incense and flowers. Having this attitude helps Karina to deal with the very real challenges of debilitation.

After telling me with some grief that her physical balance has recently declined, she tremulously read these verses from the Sufi poet Hafiz:

> *This place where you are right now*
> *God circled on a map for you.*

Wherever your eyes and arms and heart can move
Against the earth and sky,
The Beloved has bowed there—

The Beloved has bowed there knowing
You were coming . . .

After Karina finished reading the entire poem, we sat in silent appreciation. Then Karina said she had been listening to some tapes that a friend had sent her on healing and letting go of your wounds. Something in the language made her feel terrible, as though her symptoms meant she was holding on to her illness and therefore not being spiritual enough.

I responded by assuring her that her relationship to the sacred is very private and intimate, and no one else could know what is true for her. We can read or see or appreciate things that open us to the depths of the soul and touch our hearts with their beauty and poignancy. But when we take in other people's opinions in this most private area, we often find them indigestible. Instead of nourishing us, these ideas make us constrict inside, and we have to spend a tremendous amount of psychic energy just to metabolize their toxicity.

Many prevailing theories have this excruciating effect, whether from cultural, spiritual, or New Age healing ideals. Ironically, most attitudes about the body are very mental and mechanistic. Be aware of this as you note the effect of certain ideas on your inner environment; find what feeds you and weed out what feels punishing, toxic, or harsh. Embrace what allows you to breathe fully, to be spacious with yourself, and to swell open in heart, body, and soul.

THE BODY IS A MYSTERY

Our model of the body could use some revamping. The language used to describe "the body" is far too literal; internal truths are best hinted at through metaphor. Energy does not stop at the boundary of the skin; bodies are more than muscle, fat, blood, and bone. Our bodies are not just heavy old shoes we walk around in. What we call the body is a great mystery.

To shift your perception to that inquiry is a powerful way to free yourself from feeling imprisoned in the flesh.

The ideals that drive women crazy are sterile, soulless, and devoid of poetry. Enter the soul of your body and hear its poetry. Here are some alternative realities.

The Ocean of Love

The primal, creative movement of life is wave motion. There is an ocean of movement flowing around us and through us all the time. Life is movement, and we are movement; there is no separation in this oceanic dance. What is within and what is without merge in a continuous exchange, a seamless energetic flow. The beating of the heart, the waves of breath, and the streaming of blood and lymph are not isolated, internal processes, but part of the larger dance of creation. Within this embrace of movement, notions of solidity, rigidity, and isolation dissolve.

Our bodies are mostly water. Through this fluidity we resonate with the First Mother, the ocean, and the genesis of life on this planet. Our cells remember: in the womb, the growth of the embryo recapitulates the stages of evolution; the salinity of blood and amniotic fluid is the same as seawater. In many ways the sea still moves within us.

The fluid state is a healing state, a state of potentiality. When we consciously yield to this fluidity in meditation, we experience ourselves as immersed in the primordial womb, nourished and supported in an ocean of love. Swim in this ocean and be created anew.

Your Galactic Body

Our bodies are 99.99 percent space. The atoms of any body consist mostly of space, and in this vastness electrons flash, spin, appear, and disappear. We are galaxies: rich black space and scintillating points of light. Scientists speculate that most of cosmic space is "dark matter," a fertile field within which the stars take form, are born, and die. Matter, mater, mother! Matter itself is composed of elements created as long ago as the Big Bang. The calcium in our bones and the iron in our blood come from the explosive death of supernovae. Matter and energy intertwine—which is which? Enter this mystery with wonder.

MORE ABOUT MEDITATION AND SEX

Your Own Way

Embodied meditation is a key to your sensuality, and sensuality is a key to your sexuality and your power. When you enter the body, you enter your sensual nature, and issues of sexuality are bound to arise. For most of us, sex is a highly charged subject. Remember that your sensuality and sexuality are for you, first and foremost. Whether you are alone, with a man, or with a woman, meditation can enhance your eroticism—the kind that is healthful and satisfying for you.

Sexual energy, eros, creativity, life force, and the sacred are inter-changeable terms. All reflect the transformative power of the feminine that conceives, gestates, and gives birth to new life. We are erotic beings, and whether you express that in creating a family, creating art, creating a career, or falling in love with life, sexual energy is your birthright and your primal source.

Colette, a filmmaker and voice coach in her forties, reveals this link. "I often get turned on as soon as I close my eyes to meditate. For a while I thought I should give up meditating and just be good and go to church. But even in church, singing and praying, the exuberant energy excited me. I thought, 'What's wrong with me?' Eventually I realized that there is no separation between sexual and spiritual energy. This is life force. It is creation. It is how we all got here. Everybody's so busy trying to transcend and push it down. In singing, you use your sexual center, you send the energy down so that the voice is free to flow up and out. You go in both directions. When anyone is singing from deep in the body, that's God."

Learn to allow the current of eroticism to circulate through your body; be nourished and vitalized by it. Then you can choose if, how, and when to share that with another.

Let no one shame you for your body or for your sexual nature, no matter what. I know, I know—easier said than done. The voices of pressure can come from any direction: you're too much, you're not enough. There is no area of our being more vulnerable than sexuality, regardless of gender. Anybody who's been paying attention knows the challenges in sex and intimacy. But a woman's eroticism can fully blossom only in an atmosphere of relaxation, safety, and trust. Many subtle factors disturb the climate for lovemaking; the slightest emotional tension, mistrust, or unprocessed friction between partners rips the fabric of pleasure by making it almost impossible to relax.

If you are feeling disenfranchised from that source within, it may help to understand that part of what you are feeling is collective, not just personal to you. Throughout history women have endured all manner of degradation, and the violence continues to this day. To some degree every woman carries an ancestral rage and sorrow in her soul. Referring to ancient times, when female sexuality was honored and revered, Maureen Murdock writes: "Most women have lost that sense of power connected with their sexuality. Man has demeaned woman instead by calling her temptress, evil seductress, devourer. The original power of the goddess's raw sexual and procreative energy has been seen as an enormous threat to masculine authority. It has also been perceived as counterproductive to our cultural work ethic." The collective horrors of rape, incest, and physical cruelty to women are engraved in the female psyche. All too often they are personal horrors. If that is true in your life, know that you can be healed.

Our natural eroticism should be a fount of joy, not of shame or fear. That is where meditation can help. Meditation is a sanctuary for intimacy with yourself. Within its safe atmosphere you can develop your deeply personal connection to pleasure, without any demand for it to become sexualized, or for it to fulfill someone else's Hollywood fantasy. Let meditation be a place where you follow your own inner guidance and get used to what feels good to you. This is one of the best ways to heal sexual trauma. In addition, many forms of therapy address these wounds, slowly rebuilding your sense of self. Eventually you will retrieve and restore your erotic being.

Female Yang

Feminine energy is not only yin and receptive. Access to your yang expression is empowering, enlivening, and clarifying. It helps you to mobilize to create the life you want, and to do it now. It's the courage to be exposed, to extend into the world, to stand out with your desires and beliefs. You could call it a woman's phallic power. But contrary to expectation, this quality of assertion and expansion does not have to be interpreted as male.

A woman's yang can feel elemental—a ferocious force of nature like a river, wildfire, or thunderstorm. When harnessed, it's an electric, focused intensity. Sound sexual? It is.

Anatomically, the clitoris is the primary representative of this focused female yang. Sometimes in moments of sexual excitation the clitoris engorges with a desire to push, to reach out, to penetrate. No, Sigmund, this is not penis envy; it's a woman's own thrusting power. It's the woman-on-top aggression of going for it. The feeling can seem androgynous, but even that is too limiting a word. Deeper than cultural roles of male and female, and far more compelling, a woman's yang is to be celebrated as intrinsically feminine. For some women engaging this sexual force breaks a deep and terrifying taboo. We fear and hate that kind of power; it supposedly belongs to men and feels dangerous. Often it's been misused. Will I kill, rape, and pillage too?

You do not want to harm; that goes without saying. Think of yang energy as in service to life. It may sometimes feel violent, but it's the violence of breaking free. It *is* dangerous—to your own inhibitions. It does pierce a membrane—the shrink-wrap that holds you prisoner. And it kills illusions—the illusion that you are a prisoner.

Yin and yang both have a power and sensuality essential to your womanhood. Each mode is a gestalt of relationship to the universe. We need the balance of both: the spreading, dissolving receptivity of yin and the engaged, muscular urgency of yang. Just as with any of the pairs of opposites, we all tend to favor one side. Its complement, therefore, is always a source of revelation and liberation.

You can cultivate both qualities in meditation—and in sex. When you meditate in an embodied way, it can get really hot. You might get turned on—don't worry, that's a *good* thing! From the floor of your pelvis to the crown of your head, from your nipples to your knees, energy will play and stream. You can play with the energy: "Let's see, is it clitoris power today, or vulva? Highly charged and concentrated, or languid, soft, and melting? An exotic dance with some of each perhaps?" Choose your pleasure, and do with it what you will! Your skin will glow with a special luster, and your stride will be confident and free. And your relationships? They may well take on a thrilling new dimension.

Opening to Another

The more you inhabit your body and know your female power, the more you can open to the energy of another. You will have the sovereignty to receive without fear of being overpowered, invaded, or abused. How would that be possible if you are filled with yourself?

In any intimate relationship the flow of eros between partners is a deep energetic bond. This flow can be cultivated as a continual stream of nourishment and connection between you. If you are in an ongoing relationship, discovering and tending this connection strengthens your partnership.

The ancients understood cosmic energy as the perpetual erotic exchange between male and female aspects of the universe. The poetic symbolism of Tantra says it best: Shiva and Shakti are forever entwining in the divine dance of creativity and love. In this erotic union is ecstasy. Lovers can consciously join in this cosmic interplay. Though same-sex couples have their own version of this dance of opposites (translate at will), here we speak specifically to male-female partnering.

Happily married women will tell you that having a healthy sexual relationship is a key to their success. Men's ever-ready sexuality is famously different from women's, so coordinating the mating dance usually takes considerable awareness. In a good relationship we can communicate and continually learn from each other. Men take joy in giving a woman pleasure. The woman's task is to develop her eroticism for herself and show her mate what works. She can also intentionally and generously let erotic energy flow toward him.

If you love a man, love his body, no matter what its condition. Celebrate his soft penis; celebrate his moments of phallic strength. The conscious joining of the male *lingam* and the female *yoni* is a source of wonder and joy. Let meditation ready you for lovemaking. Do the "Lips-Labia" meditation; let your vulva swell to receive his male essence. Be Shakti in her divine radiance and invite Shiva into your succulent embrace.

Meditate often on all that you appreciate about the person you love. Appreciation means an increase in value, and love is a state of heightened appreciation. That men and women should honor and rejoice in each other's strengths seems only natural. Let's do our part, women. Appreciate your man!

Flying Sola

Many women are "sola," living alone by choice or fate. If you are without a sexual partner, you do not have to deny yourself that vitality and flow. There are times in life when celibacy is appropriate. But you do not have to forfeit the raptures of body and soul in being alone.

Exploring on your own is sometimes the most affirming and satisfying form of sexual expression, a union with the self. Many women who consciously choose to be celibate say that they still let sexual energy flow through them as a current of connectedness and joy. They may be "alone," but they are with themselves in a profound way, and they are in a sensuous relationship with life. They experience little erotic touches from nature—the sunlight, the wind, their hands in the soil of the garden, the brush of soft clothes on the body, the rhythm and sway of a walk. There are many pathways to delight. The rhapsody of listening to music or dancing can lead to wild Dionysian abandon, even in the privacy of your home.

In subtler realms, your sensuality can be the consummation of your relationship with the universe, with God, or the Divine Lover. In Hinduism the worship of Krishna is symbolized by passionate, illicit love, and devotees can enter rapture by meditating on and dancing erotically with the god. According to legend, while their husbands were sleeping, women would hear the call of Krishna's flute at night and sneak down to the river for ecstatic revelry. Many nuns know this secret ecstasy, though not too many will admit it. Take a meditative approach to your eroticism and you will discover just how powerful and mystical that inner connection can be.

❧ EXPLORATIONS

- When are you most comfortable in your body? When do you feel joy?
- Recall times of deep relaxation and pleasure. Remember and cultivate that state.
- When have you felt the life force coursing through your body?
- There are a hundred occasions throughout the day to care for yourself—washing your face, putting on lotion, getting dressed, scratching an itch. With what quality do you touch your body? Do you tend to poke and prod, flutter around lightly, pat yourself brusquely, or languidly stroke and caress? Bring more awareness to this touch.

&s WARM-UP: THE AFTERGLOW

Some day after lovemaking, take time to savor the afterglow. This is high-quality meditation time, so take advantage of it whenever you can. Instead of talking or jumping up to shower right away, arrange in advance to stay there for fifteen minutes or so to explore the deep and subtle sensations of pleasure. In orgasm currents of energy open up all through your body. You are thoroughly relaxed, and your nervous system is "reset," often more effectively than from a vacation. Get curious about the particular way *you* feel those currents and let them teach you about your inner world. Having ridden the current of love in relationship during sex (with a partner or with yourself), you can ride it in toward your own essence.

Sexual energy, psychic energy, and cosmic energy are very closely related; they are all expressions of the primal cosmic force that pulses through all of life. Tantric training is a school of meditation based on sexual energy; it has elaborate techniques for manipulating and heightening the energy flow. But here we'd like to point you toward noticing and valuing your own experience. There is a world of easily overlooked sensations; do any of these sound familiar?

- The changed way your skin is in contact with the air and the sheets.
- Tiny after-pulsations; tingles; an inner radiance.
- A craving to be snug and quiet and not to move.
- A powerful movement inward to identify with pure life force—becoming liquid or fire or light.

Appreciate the aesthetic quality of the sensations—the poetics of your interior world. Just by taking the time to appreciate this, a link is created between the subtle body and your brain. What imagery hints at your energy flow? For example, some women report that sexual energy feels like a serpentine undulation all through their core, and that in the afterglow from orgasm they feel residual inner waves. Others describe pulsations that radiate concentrically like bubbles from their body outward. Some say they feel like a river streaming with energy, or that they sparkle with a champagne-like effervescence. Others perceive their entire body as composed of infinite dancing particles of light, or as merging for a moment with the universe.

Let meditation be an arena for you to discover and revel in the secrets of your body, the very particular ways that life touches and moves through you.

If what you notice after lovemaking is a lack of sensation or difficulty having an orgasm, this is a time to be especially gentle with yourself. You may be experiencing a flood of emotions—grief, longing, rage, shame—and these may need to be expressed. Hold yourself close and love yourself up; place a hand on your heart and breathe. Request that your partner hold you as well. Allow the sensations and feelings of that loving embrace to be the focus of your meditation. Invite acceptance and tenderness to come into your body.

- Have you suffered about your body? What is the most painful aspect, the most distressing experience? Write about this in your journal; let it have voice. Express the very worst.
- What symptom(s) do you contend with, if any? What metaphor would describe it (them)?

• What old attitudes about your physicality are you ready to release?

❧ SKILL CIRCLE #11:
HOW TO LISTEN TO YOUR BODY

Body and *psyche* are words we use to hint at two aspects of one integrated being. Each is a particular expression of internal wisdom and intelligence. It is often through the body that your being speaks most clearly and insistently of what you require, informing you through symptoms of discomfort as well as sensations of pleasure and energy.

The body is like a dream, presenting its wisdom in symbolic language, and it does not lie. The body, like the psyche, is utterly patient and benevolent, holding information in the unconscious until we have the resources to integrate it consciously. When we are ready, memories, emotions, and intuitions arise as we listen, and we can consciously choose to learn from them. Body metaphors are eloquent and poetic expressions that reveal far more than clinical or intellectual interpretations. As you get familiar with listening to the poetry of your body, you will begin to trust the messages as keys to wholeness. Each symptom, at bottom, is saying, "Golly, I was just trying to help."

Inhabiting the Body

Take a tour of your body—a journey of awareness, touch, movement, and breath. Lightly touching with your hands is a wonderful way to bring more sensitivity to all the parts of your body. Let your position change from sitting to lying down to whatever is comfortable as you proceed.

There is healing power in your hands. Consider yourself a representative of the Divine Healer whose touch awakens and restores. When you touch or are touched with loving consciousness, a circuit of electrical energy is created and awareness is illuminated in the flesh. Take this into practice as you touch your own body with care.

In "Secret #4: Be Tender with Yourself" we spoke of the "soft inner touch" of thought. Just as it can be easier to have compassion for others than for yourself, touching your own body with love can be harder than touching someone else's. Notice the texture of your self-contact.

Consciously develop a loving and accepting "soft outer touch" with yourself as well.

Hands and Arms Let's begin with the hands themselves. Look at your hands, then begin to massage them together. Feel the skin and bones of every finger, the palm, the wrist. As you do so, think of all the things your hands do for you, how capable they are, how sensitive, flexible, and strong. Then shake your wrists to flop your hands back and forth, and when you stop, notice the tingle of increased circulation.

Now extend the circulation up into your arms by massaging each forearm, elbow, and upper arm, as gently or firmly as you like. Lift one arm and cup your hand under your armwell. (I've renamed the area formerly known as the pit.) Imagine it as a wellspring of energy and connection between your heart center and your arm. Now consider how your arms allow you to reach out from your chest to embrace, gather, lift, or push as needed. Let your touch be a kind of thank-you for all that your arms can do and how they connect you to the world.

Then relax for a moment and simply be aware of the sensations in your arms and hands. What do your arms and hands feel like? As you sense their energy flow, a visual image may come to mind that symbolizes how you feel inside.

Neck and Shoulders Let's continue up now, gently rubbing the tops of the shoulders and all around your neck. Feel the bones and muscles that allow your head to ride on top of your torso. Massage and explore, then relax and notice any tingling on the skin.

Now bring your awareness inside. As you breathe, sense and imagine the flow of energy through your throat passage. See whether you can make the breath sound as if it is coming from your throat (Ujayi breathing). Let the breath massage inside, gently releasing your throat and nourishing all the tissue, your vocal chords, your thyroid and parathyroid. (The thyroid is a butterfly-shaped gland at the base of the throat; soften inside so that its wings can spread.) As you sense the energy flow, know that you are opening the channel of your voice, your creative expression in the world.

Relax completely now and simply feel the sensations and any imagery that may come as you sense this area.

Face and Head Now delicately bring your fingertips to your face and explore the texture of the skin, flesh, and underlying bone structure. Lightly brush the entire surface of your face, including your eyelids and earlobes. As you touch each area, appreciate its function: your eyes, ears, nostrils, cheeks, and lips, your eyebrows and forehead. Thank your face for not only seeing, hearing, smelling, speaking, and eating but for being able to express feelings with such a wide range of nonverbal clues.

Now let your fingers massage up into your scalp, all around your ears, and over the base of your skull. Tug gently on your hair (if this feels good). Then relax and enjoy the increased circulation around your head.

Bring your attention inside with your eyes softly relaxed and closed. Imagine that your brain floats restfully inside your head. Thank your brain for its magnificent intelligence, the myriad and intricate functions it performs whether you're awake or asleep. Feel your entire head relaxing. If you are sitting, just let it bobble on top of your spine; if you are lying down, release its weight into the floor. Without straining to find one, let any image float into your awareness. Breathe with that before going on.

Feet, Legs, and Haunches Now shift your attention all the way down to your feet and let them wiggle a bit. Bring your hands into play again, touching the skin of the sole, the arch and heel, each toe, the top of the foot and ankle. Massage each foot with the quality of pressure you like, increasing the awareness and circulation. Relax for a moment and enjoy the residual sensations in your feet. Let any image come.

Now massage up each leg into your calves and shins, around your knees, up your thighs. Spend as long as you like—there's a lot to explore. Relax each leg as you massage it so you can feel the soft texture of the muscles, the skin, and the bony support structure within. As you get to your haunches—your lower hips and thighs—appreciate the power of those big muscles and bones. Bring the love of your hands into your entire leg, including the protective layers of fat. (If you notice a twinge inside at the mention of the "f" word, take a few conscious breaths to flush that feeling out and replace it with kindness.)

Now plant the soles of your feet on the ground and let them take some of your weight. If you are lying down, bend your knees and press into your feet as though to lift your hips; let your pelvis hover slightly if comfortable. If sitting, you could come to standing. Shift your weight through each foot, and feel your muscles engage. Begin to contemplate the many ways your legs support you, connect you to the ground, and propel you through the activities of your day. Take a minute, either standing or reclining, to play with the movement and any imagery that arises from the connection in your legs and feet.

Your Sacred Sacrum Now come to a sitting position and bring your hands to the back of your pelvis. The sacrum is a wide triangular bone, with the coccyx (tailbone) as the downward point. The tailbone is a vestigial reminder of our creaturehood, so take a moment to appreciate your animal roots.

Gently massage through the sacrum and the surrounding flesh of the hips; press your thumbs into the little valleys of the bone and along the downward slopes of the triangle, which are your sacroiliac joints. Now just rest your hands there and slightly rock your pelvis forward and back and feel its subtle movement. Pause, relax your arms, and sit for a moment sensing the area at the base of your spine.

Then ease yourself onto your back with your knees bent and feet flat on the floor, your hips relaxed and heavy into the ground. From your tailbone to your lower ribs is a natural arch—the lumbar curve. As you exhale, gently bring that area toward the floor, relaxing again to neutral as you inhale. After a few breaths, begin to explore different ways to tilt your pelvis and nuzzle your lower back into the ground. As always, this should feel good; if it doesn't, either stop or adjust so that it does.

Then relax for several breaths. The downward pointing triangle of the sacrum is esoterically related to Shakti energy, or the female aspect of life force. Breathe into that sacred triangle and enjoy that connection.

Belly Now massage gently all around your abdomen. Explore in a circular pathway—from your lower belly up under your right ribs, across your solar plexus to your left ribs, down to your left pubis and across to the right. Then bring your hands to rest on your lower belly. As you breathe, notice the swell of the breath under your hands—rising as you inhale, sinking back down as you exhale. Feel how the breath massages everywhere inside, cleansing and nourishing all your internal organs: liver, gallbladder, spleen, stomach, pancreas, kidneys, adrenals, intestines, uterus, bladder. Think of all the organs pulsing with life energy as they do their part to take care of your whole body. Take a moment to thank them.

Dr. Geeta Iyengar, daughter of the yoga master B. K. S. Iyengar, says that in modern women the uterus tends to be hard because of stress, which challenges our hormonal balance. Allowing that area to be soft is important, especially during the years before and during menopause. Imagine the womb floating softly inside the belly with lots of room to breathe.

Pause now and simply enjoy the breath, warmth, and connection in your belly. Rest for several moments with this awareness, and again, if an image comes, spend some time acknowledging it.

Breasts Staying on your back, gently massage up the front and sides of your chest. As you approach your breasts, move slowly and give them special care. Pause and let your hands cradle your breasts in some way, taking in the warmth and flow of contact. Feel the movement beneath your hands as your lungs fill and release. Let your awareness penetrate deep into your chest and imagine your heart energy suffusing each breast. Again, you may receive a visual image as well, so take several minutes to breathe with all these impressions.

Full Body Become aware of the back of the heart center and let it melt back into the floor. Bring your attention to the breadth of your back and hips as they contact the ground. Then gently extend your legs, if that is comfortable, and scan the back surface of your body from your heels to your head.

Spend several minutes letting your attention flow freely through your entire body—front, back, sides, from within all the way out through your skin. The membrane of the skin is an interface between the inner and outer worlds. Recognize what a marvelous container the skin is—how it envelops the whole package that is your body. Receive these impressions of your full form—what I call "global body awareness." Is there an image that would hint at this full body experience?

As you scan this way, your attention may be drawn to certain areas of more sensation—increased tingling, warmth, tightness, pain, some kind of internal tug. These are little signals from places that may have something special to communicate—energy that wants to reconnect with the whole. You can choose to give these parts more attention, continuing with the following suggestions. Consider this localized attention a body version of the saying "Think globally, act locally."

Let a Symptom Speak

You can relate to a body part or symptom as an inner character and receive its metaphorical gift. Beginning with one of the images you discovered earlier, or with the sensations that you are experiencing now. See "Secret #8: Say Yes to Every Part of Yourself," especially the "Inner Theater" skill circle, to refresh your understanding of characters and how to work with them.

"Become" the part in your imagination and allow it to speak to you—that is, to your central witnessing self. Write in your journal as the voice of the symptom; let it communicate its needs, feelings, or insights.

Draw the feeling tone of the symptom or part of your body. Your earlier impressions from "Inhabit Your Body" can come onto your page—in color, shape, and quality of movement. You can also draw by letting go of any preconceived image and give over to the energetic quality and emotion. Let your hand choose the color and then dance with it on the paper.

Bring actual movement of some kind (and do be kind) into that part of your body and notice the heightened sensations. How does its energy want to move? What are its qualities? What are its emotions? You may not get concrete answers, but the spontaneous communication within the movement can be thoroughly eloquent.

Now ponder these explorations. What metaphor have they revealed? What does it express? In what way can you honor that message from your body and psyche?

Body Poem

An elegant way to acknowledge the expressions from your body is to create a simple poem. As you bring awareness to every part within the whole, you may find that a word or two naturally drifts into your mind. Write them down, and then play with how they may link together in surprising ways. You could put each word or phrase on an index card and scramble them around. Or arrange them together in an aesthetically pleasing order.

This is wonderful to do in a group or with a friend. Speak your body poem out loud, with the feeling that is laced within the words. Let the power, beauty, and poignancy of your body's poetry be felt and heard.

Get Help If You Need It

We are fortunate in our time to have many resources for working with the body. Massage therapy or other bodywork, dance therapy or movement classes can all give you an arena for direct physical exploration. In addition, many psychotherapists, especially those with a Jungian or archetypal background, can provide tools and insights into the metaphorical and emotional messages from your body and psyche.

Sometimes physical pain is a cry for medical attention, so heed that message if you get it. Holistic practitioners treat the symptom within the context of your whole being, but there are also times when you may opt for standard allopathic treatment (which often addresses only the symptom). Just remember that the larger, global embrace of loving awareness is primary, and cultivate that for yourself over time. Do not hesitate to enlist help; we all need assistance and companionship along the way.

❧ MEDITATIONS

The Great Mother's Love

How we relate to our bodies and the feminine has a great deal to do with Mother, and whether our association is positive or negative. Even if the relationship to our biological mother leaves something to be desired, we can "re-mother" ourselves in consciousness and claim the birthright of our cosmic home.

Whether we are aware of it or not, we are always in the arms of the Great Mother. Our bodies are of Her body, the fecund body of Nature in which we live and move and have our being. In this meditation, you bring consciousness to this most basic relationship. Experience breath, gravity, pulsation, light, color, shape, and movement as gifts of life to you.

Begin by sitting comfortably with your eyes open. Bring your awareness to the simple sensory impressions around you. Notice the quality of light and the variety of colors in the objects you see. Soften your eyes and let them drink in nourishment from those hues. Is there any movement within your visual range? What blend of activity and stillness do you see? What sounds do you hear? What pleasure can you find in these impressions? Take several minutes to recognize yourself as immersed within this texture of life. (At some point your eyes may want to close, so let them open and close naturally as you proceed.)

Now bring your attention to your breath. Breath is fluid. The ocean of air around us is fluid, flowing everywhere over the earth and seas. It is the breath of the Great Mother. As you breathe, feel how the flow of breath draws you into deeper connection with all of nature. Imagine that with each breath you receive Her love into every part of your body.

Begin to sense your physicality—the shape, density, and texture of matter. Become aware of gravity and how your weight rests on the vast body of Earth. What sensations inform you of that relationship? Our planet is flying through space at unimaginable speed, but we are held to its surface, safe and sound in apparent stillness. Feel how gravity holds you from below like a huge hug, and let yourself drop into that foundation. Imagine your body as inextricably part of the larger terrestrial body; soften the edges, the mental boundary between you and the natural world. Notice how every sense impression is actually an intimate touch from some aspect of life.

When you realize that your body is not separate and isolated from nature, how does it change how you feel inside? What is it to be in your body? As you ponder these impressions, various thoughts, associations, and emotions are likely to surface. Some of them may be painful, cynical, angry, or sad. Accept them and hear them all, no matter what they say. Know that they are coming into the embrace of awareness to be healed. They are coming out of hiding and into the presence of love.

Suffuse your entire body with this loving consciousness. Use the touch of awareness and your hands to channel healing and care. Spend extra time with any particular place that is calling for more attention, through sensations of either pleasure or discomfort; you may have a symptom you're dealing with, or internal imagery, or simple curiosity about some physical experience. Use the suggestions f m the skill circle to address any of these calls.

To relax into the larger body is a profound release. As the illusions of isolation melt away, tears may come too. The tears may have an emotional quality, or they may simply be a physiological release—your body letting go. Each time you meditate with body awareness, the connection will grow stronger and more accessible. Be patient with yourself; be kind. Your consciousness is unfolding inexorably, and healing happens in its own good time.

The Floating World

This meditation about sublime immersion in the ocean of love is especially soothing with gentle music. Create a soft and warm space on the floor and lie down on your back in luxury. Put a cushion under your knees to relieve your lower back if you like, and perhaps a soft pillow under your head. You want to feel completely safe, warm, and comfortable.

Step 1 Take several minutes to lie back and relax. Let your weight release downward and your back spread open into the ground, as if your entire body is thawing like ice cream in the sun. Become aware of this paradox: the more you give in to your weight, the lighter you feel. Enjoy the sensations of melting and floating free. Dissolve into flow.

Step 2 Keeping your hands as relaxed as can be, bring your awareness to the very tips of your fingers. Begin to move them in the smallest possible way. Curve your fingertips in ever so slightly and release them back out. Spread them apart with the subtlest micro-movements and feel the webbing between your fingers stretch like gossamer fabric. Notice another paradox: the tiniest movement is a doorway that opens up a universe of sensation. Stay with this as long as you like, releasing into this soft and spacious awareness.

Step 3 Shift your attention to your toes. In the same way, find little movements there. Wiggle each toe; spread them apart gently. Continue, softly moving energy through your feet.

As you bring subtle movement to your extremities in this gentle way, your whole body spreads softly and extends wide. Other parts of your body may begin to move in subtle waves. Keep giving over to this fluid and spacious relaxation. You may feel as though you are weightlessly suspended among the stars, floating in the cosmic sea, or immersed in a warm and nurturing womb. Enter the ocean of love and surrender to its tender support.

We suggest doing this meditation after the "Spine Wave" stretch (page 267) or the "Sway Away" meditation (in "Secret #4: Be Tender with Yourself"). The larger wave motion of the torso in those movements instills undulations in your body that you can take into the subtle mode of sensing here.

❧ GOING FURTHER

Lips-Labia Meditation

In this meditation, you revel in the sensuality, softness, and mobility of your lips. There is a resonance between the lips of the face and those of the vulva; neuromuscularly and poetically, the two mouths are intimately related. How this is true for you is an ongoing discovery.

Let's begin with the upper lips. As you bring your attention to your mouth, relax your tongue and jaw. Feel the shape of your lips; begin to gently pucker into a kiss and then release. Slowly open and close your mouth into a large "O," spread your lips into a smile, and then soften again. Explore delicate pulsing nuances of movement. If you like, bring your fingers to your lips and sense their texture. Place your fingertips inside the soft, moist flesh. Appreciate the beauty and sensuousness of your mouth.

Now shift your attention to your vulva. Can you see your labia in your mind's eye? What sensations are you aware of? If you are sitting, feel the contact of the floor of your pelvis with the seat. Begin to explore the sense of movement, little contractions of the labia and inside the vagina. I've never been fond of the term "Kegels"—it's so clinical, and who wants someone else's name down there? The yogis call these exercises "mulabandha"—not much better. But the toning action of drawing up the pelvic floor provides marvelous support for the female organs, the bladder, and (praise be) fuller orgasms. A client once suggested calling this exercise "The Anemone," which I love because it refers both to a beautiful flower and to a diaphanous creature that pulses its way in the sea. So instead of a medical prescription, think of the labial movement as a lush and poetic event. Cultivating the aesthetics of sensuality opens up your inner body like nothing else.

Continue now by adding the anemone-like movement through your mouth. As your attention flows back and forth through the labia and the lips, you may feel the inner channel between them opening and energy undulating through your core. Take your time to enjoy.

These sensations are obviously erotic and stimulating, a kind of lovemaking with yourself. Use this to become even more intimate with your personal pathways of delight. It can prepare you to blossom more deeply with your lover or take you into a luscious dream. The air itself may shape-change, like Eros, into a perfect caress, the invisible arms of your Lover Divine.

The Galactic Body Meditation

There is an ancient esoteric saying, "As above, so below." Science seems to be confirming this truth. Consider that your body is mostly "empty" space. Just as the distance between stars is inconceivably vast, so too the spaciousness within an atom is incomprehensibly great. What appears to be solid and heavy is actually infinitesimal vibration between subatomic particles with almost no physical dimension or weight, and vast distances between them. The movement of matter is as subtle and refined as a thought.

We are privileged to live in an era of technology that can directly descry the immensity of the cosmos. We have all seen photographs of the majestic swirl of galaxies. Cosmologists have determined that there are 400 billion stars in our galaxy alone, and 50 billion galaxies in the known universe. The mind boggles, but as we contemplate such boundlessness, consciousness makes a giant leap.

What is your favorite image of space? Meditate on the spaciousness of your body, and let your imagination take flight. Can you imagine the galactic glory of your body? Can you imagine yourself being as limitless as the night sky?

Realize that your essence is not confined within the boundary of your skin. Give your awareness infinite space. You don't have to cramp your thoughts inside your skull; let them float out from your head. Imagine your essence stretching out to the stars, expanding like the universe itself.

The substance of the stars shines in every cell that is you. Ponder the mystery of this reality.

A star expands, explodes, and dies in an orgasmic supernovan flash.
Elements are birthed in its white-hot fire . . .
Atoms split and fuse into molecules, zooming through galactic space.
They are here: this Earth is stardust, this body, yours . . .
Infinite tiny particles of light pulsing softly,
Like a million tiny dragons everywhere—

Undulating, vibrant, multicolored prisms—
All matter imbued with consciousness,
With light, with love . . .

&ab &ab &ab

&ab REFLECTIONS

- What new appreciation of your body can you cultivate?
- After exploring a symptom, what message have you discovered in it?
- What new ways can you nourish yourself?
- What are some simple ways to love yourself throughout the day? What special pleasures can you allow? Commit to one daily act.

SECRET #12
LIVE IT UP

Ah, lots of creative energy today, lots to give . . .
I will meditate with excitement about life,
In gratitude and wonder that I even exist . . .

So many billions of years ago the universe burst into being:
The Big Bang, the primordial shout of creation.
Light began to shine in countless stars,
Space itself began to blossom into infinity,
And dark matter gave birth to us all . . .

All matter is singing, vibrating with that primal pulse,
The O, the Om, the sacred sound . . .

I sit in the richness called silence,
My internal strings struck by chords of awe—
That evolution created such possibility:
This dance, this song, this moment of life we share.
Let me play my part in the symphony . . .
Let me join the harmony!

I hear the "Ooooo," clear like a bell, rising through my core.
The mantra emanates in all directions . . .
Concentric rings of "O" radiate out from my center in waves,
Spreading the sound of love around the globe—
Creating space, creating relationship, creating touch.

I plunge into the "O" like a pebble in a pond.
I send my essence out, I give myself away . . .

My chest lifts full, breathes open and free.
My heart shines through my head, my belly, my feet.
This is the power of "O," the joy of creation
As I sing my song back to the stars.

THE CALL TO RETURN

Meditation and expression are complementary. Just as there is a rhythm that calls you into meditation to renew yourself, so there is a call to return to the world to put the energies you've invoked into play. It is the swing of the pendulum, and the further you go in one direction, the further you go in the other. Meditation is preparation for life; it is as much about expressing yourself as it is about resting in yourself. It is in your activity, in your work and your relationships, that the most interesting benefits show up.

Be open to and welcome all desires, for each leads you into the self as well as out into action. Desire is a current of electricity that connects inner and outer, so within desire is your path of integration—the yoga of everyday life. We are social creatures. We need to be social, and it's good for our health in every way. Exercise your socializing instinct when you meditate; cultivate and celebrate your love for the world.

Meditation can generate a sense of simmering in passion and excitement about your life; always accept this response and breathe deeply with it when it happens. Let the desires you have cherished during meditation take you back out to live your passion. The purpose of meditation is to link your inner resources to the whole process of fulfilling desire—the action of creativity. Your ultimate criterion for assessing how well meditation is working in your life lies in the answer to this question: what does it give to your everyday life, to your ability to handle yourself in the world, and to your ability to live the way you want to?

One of the marvelous long-range effects of this integrative approach is a new perception of the whole fabric of your life—the warp and woof of all its challenges and pain. You begin to sense a larger design—an inevitability or purpose behind your personal history, and with this awareness comes forgiveness. All your circumstances and choices are illuminated as necessary experiences in becoming who you are today. You come to realize and accept what is yours to be and do—the fulfill-ment of this design. Willingly, humbly, eagerly, you take your place within the colorful tapestry of life.

MENTAL REHEARSAL

One of the arts of meditating is learning to tolerate excitement and to breathe with your bliss. You are building a bridge between the depths of your inner life and the details of daily action.

Thinking through and rehearsing future actions is a natural aspect of the meditative process. The body goes into relaxation and then pre-views the attitudes and muscle movements of upcoming challenges and rehearses the most efficient and effective ways to respond. When thoughts about future activities arise, you may not only allow them but also intentionally focus on them. A mental rehearsal helps to remove excess tension and anxiety about performance. Athletes all over the world do this in preparation for their events. Meditation is tuning your-self up to excel, to thrive and be in harmony in your life. Figure that half your meditation time will be spent tuning up this way.

In meditation you are able to relax into urgency. When you begin to think about your everyday life, what you're really doing is getting prac-tice in staying relaxed while doing whatever is on your mind. You can track every detail of your excitement, every thump of your heart in anx-iety, hope, and fear, but because you are only sitting there and "rehears-ing," the anxiety is massaged out of your system.

Let meditation help you get ready for important events. If some-thing is coming up—a presentation, a request for a raise, a crucial talk with someone you love—you will find yourself rehearsing it during meditation. Allow this. Then, to your surprise, you will function better because you are prepared, more poised, and at ease. Ease in action is grace—an economy and naturalness of movement. There is no extrane-ous motion, no waste of energy or distraction, as witnessed in many athletes and animals. In meditation you learn grace under fire and how to move through your life like a gazelle.

THE CREATIVE URGE

Meditation is creative. It is like giving birth to and nurturing your future self, the self you will become. Your emotional body is being stretched and strengthened so that you'll have the courage to live fully. Sometimes you will be in a creative fervor during meditation. Enjoy the feeling. You are building not only your dreams and inspirations but the emotional resilience to sustain those dreams. Sometimes you will experience healing imagery. When you meditate, any energy that is stuck will loosen up and start to flow. You may be flooded with creative ideas. Learn to accept new sensations of movement, new impulses emerging for manifestation in your life.

The meditative state is famous for eliciting unexpected revelations. Whether in the art of your life or in a specific creative project, it is often when we let go of the problem that the solution intuitively appears. Creating is not about control, but about sensing what wants to happen and participating with that movement. This is mastery. Your creativity is a flow that cannot be forced—but it can be tended. When you are in the creative streaming of your own life, you sense that "yes, this feels right," even or especially when it is challenging.

Live *your* life, the quality and expression that you are designed for. You are the author of your life; claim this authority. Do what is yours to do, contribute what is yours to give. There may be no greater satisfaction.

Meditation for the World

The sanctuary of meditation provides an embrace big enough for all the love you have in your heart that sometimes is too powerful, too vast, to express to another human being. In meditation you can let yourself give over to all the passion, compassion, and empathy that you feel. Your cares and concerns can be transmuted into a conscious blessing for loved ones, for humanity, for the planet. In this way, whatever you experience—all your joy and suffering—can be seen as a gift of relatedness that takes you into deeper connection with the world.

Meditation for the Planet Women are empathetic and always at least vaguely aware of the suffering in the world. Sometimes we can take specific actions, and sometimes there is nothing outward that can be done.

In such cases, it helps to find an inward way to address the situation, so that our energy doesn't get stuck in the pain.

In meditation you can breathe with awareness of the situation and send your energy and love out to that place in the world, or to the planet as a whole.

First spend several minutes establishing your own ground. Recognize your inner strength, your capacity to love, your connection to humanity and the earth. Each time you inhale, draw in the power of love, until you feel it pulsing fully within you.

Then, when you are ready, bring more attention to your exhalation. As your breath flows out, send something of your essence out with it. Join with the situation and reach out to it in your awareness. Give it your breath and consciousness. Let healing energy flow through your heart.

Taking action in this inner, energetic way can relieve some of your frustration and despair over circumstances beyond your control.

Sometimes you will also realize in meditation that there is some small outward action you can take. Every little bit counts.

LUCY'S LARGESSE

Lucy is a writer in her early fifties who has practiced meditation for about twelve years. "Speed and doing too much is unwise, at least for me. I make mistakes, and sometimes I hurt people. The antidote to a life that has too much in it is to sit daily. I can be with what is really going on. I have a moment to see how I am, and to sense it.

"All my senses are involved. I feel my breath, I hear the outside sounds, I see the light in the room. There's a pleasurable sense of going down, as if my center of gravity is dropping down. Then I know I'm letting go. It feels like there is a lake inside, and that I am *deeply home*. From that place could come generosity and wisdom. It is no accident that there is the term 'being centered.' When I meditate I touch into the physical truth of that. I can notice if I'm leaning forward, rushing and pushing in fear to make something happen. When I am resting in my center, the whole inner channel opens. I am there with every part of myself—my grief, my folly, my longing, my love.

"One of the great gifts of meditation practice is that it enabled me to be larger than I thought I was. It enabled me to do work in the world, to alleviate some suffering, and to go beyond my own needs. That has been a blessing, and I hope to find that again and again throughout my life."

✌ SANDRA'S JOBS

Sandra is thirty-six, newly married, and in the first years of her profession as a therapist. "There is so much happening for me these days. Meditation gives me time to reflect upon the depth that runs through all the different areas of my life. I take time to feel the things that are my job to do, in every sense of the word. I meditate on my clients, the members of my family and friends, and the life I am creating together with my husband. When I tune in to myself, I notice a trembling inside before the awesomeness of it all.

"Sometimes I scare myself off from meditating, if I make it into an obligation. I know it is a way to stay in touch with my potential, with the bigness of what wants to come. When I think about the bigness, I get overwhelmed. Throughout my life I've put obligation into learning and accomplishing. I can make my job seem so heavy, as if I have to bear down. So I've had to learn that meditation can be more forgiving, more formless . . . that it is not about trying so hard or achieving.

"As a kid, time was a lot more lazy. I remember sitting near the window in the sun on Sunday mornings—a suspended feeling of just enjoying myself. So that's the state that I cultivate now. I like to meditate lying down in the morning, staying languid but aware for about half an hour. I also like to write every day, similar to the "morning pages" from *The Artist's Way*. Lately I've started taking Tuesday mornings when I'm alone to have the space to move in a contemplative way, give over to all the currents that are flowing inside me. I need the solitude and silence to stay grounded and to remember the forgiveness."

Stretch into Life

You may discover that you have more life in you than you know how to express. Sometimes after meditation you can feel all dressed up with no place to go. This is because you are living at a new level of energy and perceptiveness that you're not yet used to, or perhaps the circumstances of your life haven't quite caught up with the new you. This is always a challenge.

Through meditation you will get hunches for new activities and even dreams you'd given up on, but use daring to follow through on them. You may feel fear of expressing yourself or of expanding out into the world. If you have experienced profound disappointment, it may take some time to adjust to the possibility of fulfillment. This is both exciting and totally terrifying. You can learn to love again. You can return to life.

Whenever we start to use some long-neglected faculty, it's a bit like when your foot has been asleep and there is intolerable tingling as circulation is restored. Expect this to be uncomfortable and know that eventually it will work its way through. Here again, the art is to allow the process and tolerate these new sensations. Your body and psyche will gradually adapt to the more expansive energies, and soon you'll be able to take the action you crave.

❧ ALICE'S HEART

In an interview with Sharon Salzberg, Alice Walker said: "You know what hearts are for? Hearts are there to be broken, and I say that because that seems to be just part of what happens with hearts. I mean, mine has been broken so many times that I have lost count. But it just seems to be broken open more and more and more, and it just gets bigger. In fact, I was saying to my therapist not long ago, 'You know, my heart by now feels open like a suitcase. It feels like it has just sort of dropped open, you know, like how a big suitcase just falls open. It feels like that.'

"Instead of that feeling of having a thorn through your heart, that feeling Pema Chodron talks about in tonglen meditation, you have a sense of openness, as if the wind could blow through it. And that's the way I'm used to my heart feeling. The feeling of the heart being so open that the wind blows through it. I think that is the way it's supposed to feel when you're in balance. And when you get out of balance, you feel like there's no wind, there's no breeze, there's just this rock, and it has a big thing sticking through it. I don't know how you get from one feeling to the other, except through meditation, often, but also activism, just seeing what needs to be done in the world, or in our families, and just start doing it."

Alice Walker has always followed her inner guidance, taking up issues in her writing that alienated many people in her community. "My little theory is that you find that you just keep doing the thing that gets you kicked out, and this has everything to do with living as your true self. And then you meet up with all the other people who've been kicked out. And then you have your team, and it's a team of everybody. I definitely feel that way. I feel that because of the positions I have taken and the things that I have written, I often find myself totally out. But it never means that I'm alone, because then I discover that there are all these other people who also have subversive thoughts and have also done and written things that their particular clan didn't approve of. And so there we all are, and there begins to be built a whole other community, a whole other family of people who are not related by color, blood, sex, or whatever, but by vision. That's how I feel, that I'm a part of a whole community of great people, and it's not about race, it's about vision and what we think the world will be and should be."

GATHER TWO OR MORE

Often we think of meditation as a retreat, a pause or interlude between activities. But sometimes it seems like the best contact we ever get with the world. Harmony takes over, and we are completely at home within ourselves and our environment. Horizons expand, and we awaken to the vastness and beauty of the earth. The thought strikes: this is reality, this is the real world.

Meditating with others stretches this perception. Even with just one other person, a thicker field of energy is created that supports the shared silence, especially when there is strong rapport among you. When couples, families, or friends meditate together, you engage in a silent conversation about what harmony is. Individuality finds its place within the whole and merges with infinity. It is social, like sharing a meal, but you are being fed at a different restaurant, feasting on concoctions of air, light, sound, and feeling. A sense of community strengthens this awareness. In church, for example, people often enter the richness of silence in between the prayers and sermons and songs.

Meditating together creates a peaceful bonding. Because meditation is undemanding time, it has a freeing, intimate quality similar to when people are alone with their pets. Meditation cuts through the shyness and awkwardness, the limitation of words. In ordinary social discourse moments of shared silence happen spontaneously, but people are usually embarrassed by silence and tend to fill it. So it is wonderful to intentionally make time to dwell with each other in that easy flow.

Consider meeting with your lover, friends, or family once a week to meditate. Use this book for ideas—read, discuss, contemplate, move, and breathe. Get to know each other at that deep silent level, and you will create an unshakable foundation for enduring relationships.

BREATHE IN YOUR OWN ATMOSPHERE

All of the meditations in this book will lead you to an embodied experience of your essential nature. When you learn to live from what you love, it is as though you carry your own atmosphere with you wherever you go. As you bask in the pleasure of your senses and your deep feminine instincts, you create a nourishing substance to draw from throughout the day. Your inner being blooms, and you begin to emanate a special essence that others can appreciate—your unique personal scent. Breathe in your own fragrant atmosphere. Spread it around. Love it, glory in it—with no apology and no shame!

Break Those Taboos

- Be happy.
- Be glorious.
- Be wild.
- Be sensuous.
- Laugh a lot.
- Take time for yourself.
- Say no to what you don't want.
- Say what you do want.
- Find your own style.
- Be different.
- Don't apologize for being yourself.
- Say what you see.
- Do what you love.

✖ EXPLORATIONS

- On what occasion were you the most excited you've ever been in your life?
- When have you experienced disappointment? Did the loss dampen your enthusiasm and confidence? Did it lead you into compassion? What happened to your joy? Where does your joy emerge now?
- What makes you laugh? What friends, movies, cartoons, or comedians tickle your funny bone? When do you laugh at yourself?
- Write about your passion. What do you care most about?
- If you imagine yourself in your life completely expressive and free, what do you see? What desires want to be lived out? What are your dreams?

&s SKILL CIRCLE #12: HOW TO MEDITATE IN THE MOVEMENT OF A DAY

Enter by Any Gate

Each of us can have our own menu of meditations that we cycle through, a handful of favorite ways to connect inside. Create your own menu of meditations that you love. Together they reflect your whole self in this moment. Each meditation satisfies some part of you, providing a nutritional element that is required just as much as vitamin C, water, or protein. On any particular day one or more may be called for.

As you respond to the needs of your life and to your desires, select the mode of meditating that works the best each day. As women, we can't have just one monotonous meditation; we need a variety to choose from, like different textures, colors, or styles. Always feel free to improvise! We have given you many secrets and many ways of responding to your body and its rhythms. One chapter may have particular relevance for you, and its secret could be a doorway into that day's meditation. Learn to respond to the call for that tone of meditation and to enter by its secret gate.

The needs and rhythms of each day determine the structure of your meditation—the kind of meditation you do, how long you meditate, and where. For example, when I am working on performances, I allow extra time to meditate because I'll be so busy reviewing the choreography or text. To prepare on the day of a performance I make sure to give myself an afternoon meditation to dwell in the atmosphere I want to create.

Once in 1969 Lorin picked up a seminar leader at the airport and took him to the university to teach during the day. "After he was finished in the late afternoon, I asked him if he wanted me to take him to a restaurant in the airport, and he said he wanted to go someplace where he could meditate. I said, 'Do you have time? You have to get on a plane.' And he said, 'I don't have time not to meditate. In my job, I can't afford not to be at my best.'"

Menu of All Meditations

Below is a list of all the meditations we have offered in this book. The ones that are starred (*) are great to do as one- to five-minute mini-meditations throughout the day. Some days you may feel like sitting quietly; other times you may want to move or be outside. And sometimes you simply must lie down. Even a minute can refresh, remind, and empower you. Over time your menu of meditations may change, or you will want to add more as you unfold in awareness, including more parts of yourself. Becoming whole means embracing all aspects of who you are—a wondrous, mysterious, inclusive process!

1. Build your foundation in pleasure and bathe in the senses with:
   - The Sensuousness of Breath*
   - Music to Your Ears
   - *Mmmm* Meditation
   - Active Pleasure Meditation*
   - Favorite Sin Meditation*
   - The Secret Smile

2. Tend to your creaturehood and follow your instincts with:
   - The Elixir of Life*
   - Natural Wonder Meditation*
   - The Movement of No*
   - The Earth Circuit
   - Healing Meditation
   - Creature Meditations

3. Inhabit space fully and reclaim your power with:
   - Core Breath
   - Meditation on Sovereignty*
   - Gathering Power*
   - "I AM" Awareness
   - The Tree of Life
   - The Many-Armed Goddess

4. Soften into compassion and flow with:
   - Breath of Compassion*
   - A Gentle Awakening
   - Heart in Hand

- Soft Touch*
- Sway Away*
- The Sweetness of Space

5. Take refuge with:
   - Meditation on Giving and Receiving*
   - The Sanctuary of Your Personal Space*
   - Hum into Your Heart
   - Bathe in Light*
   - Your Secret Prayer*

6. Honor a longing or desire with:
   - Longing for the Divine
   - The Call of the Wild
   - Welcome All Desires
   - Heart's Desire Meditation

7. Respond to your body rhythms with:
   - Breath as Birth and Death
   - Bloodline
   - Umbilicus Mundi
   - The Chrysalis

8. Loosen the grip of a mood or emotion and call upon an inner ally with:
   - The Pendulum
   - Jazz Breath*
   - Behind the Mask*
   - What a Character!*
   - Yakitty-Yak, You Can Talk Back*

9. Let go into being simple with:
   - Breath Meditation: No Demands*
   - Gratitude Meditation*
   - Meditation with Earth, Air, Water, and Fire

10. Consciously excavate the depths of your soul with:
    - The Breath Beyond
    - Belly to the Ground*

- Down to the Bone Meditation
- Descent to the Goddess Meditation
- Egyptian Pose

11. Take care of a physical symptom or enter the mystery of the body with:
    - The Great Mother's Love*
    - The Floating World
    - Lips-Labia Meditation
    - The Galactic Body Meditation

12. Percolate in passion for your life and prepare to meet the world with:
    - Open your Arms to Life*
    - Let Your Sound Go Forth
    - Meditation for the World
    - The Figure 8 Movement Meditation*
    - At Home in the Universe

Recipes and Remedies

Feel free to mix and match to create your own recipe. Spend five minutes with each part. Here are some suggestions for when you are experiencing:

FEAR OR ANXIETY
Create: "Sanctuary" (page 103)
Body ritual: "Thumbs Up" (page 112)
Mantra: "Kwan Yin Mantra" (page 123)
Breath: "Breath of Compassion" (pages 98–99)
Image: "Earth Circuit" (pages 43–44)

FATIGUE
Create: "Simplicity" (page 202)
Body ritual: "Belly to the Ground" (pages 219–220)
Breath: "Elixir of Life" (page 42)
Movement: "Stretch It Out" (pages 266–268)

DEPRESSION
Create: "Sovereignty" (page 75)
Body ritual: "Dark Eyes" (page 217)
Breath: "Breath as Birth and Death" (pages 165–66)
Image: "Descent to the Goddess" (pages 222–223)
Movement: "The Sweetness of Space" (page 100)

ANGER
Create: "Your Inner Theater" (page 187)
Body ritual: "The Movement of No" (pages 42–43)
Mantra: "Kali Mantra" (page 123)
Breath: "Core Breath" (pages 74–75)
Image: "What a Character!" (pages 192–93)

SLEEPLESSNESS
Create: "A Nest" (page 39)
Body ritual: "Egyptian Pose" (page 223)
Mantra: "Your Secret Prayer" (page 129)
Breath: "The Breath Beyond" (page 219)

ILLNESS
Create: "Inner Sanctuary" (page 120)
Body ritual: "Listen to Your Body" (page 239)
Breath: "Healing Meditation" (page 44)
Image: "Rest in the Elements" (page 206)

Move Through Your Day

Here are some suggestions for how to move through the day with sensuous meditative awareness.

Waking Up Take several minutes to let yourself drift up from dreamland. If possible, do not use an alarm. Lie there within the sleepy comfort of the bed and let your senses adjust to the idea of getting up. Remember your dreams, and if you have time later, write them down.

Bless your loved ones. Feel everything you are grateful for. Do "A Gentle Awakening" ("Secret #4: Be Tender with Yourself"). Stretch a little, massage your eyes gently, and take a few breaths. Then slowly ooze out of bed and into your day.

Eating Take time before eating to savor the smell and visual appeal of your food. Prepare your senses for the pleasure of eating; get all your juices flowing. In your mind, imagine and appreciate how and where the food was grown. Find your own way to say "grace." When you take each bite, give yourself that extra second or two to savor the nuances of taste and texture. When you finish, take another few minutes to relax and digest before you jump up.

Nighttime Reflection As you get into bed at night, take a few minutes to review your day. Bask in the moments you enjoyed. If you check for unexpressed impulses and honor them, you will probably sleep better because you have tracked all those unfinished movements that usually haunt us in the night. Suggest to yourself that you will remember your dreams. Then, as you fall asleep, bless your loved ones and drift into your dreams with that fullness in your heart.

For better sleep, start to slow down an hour or so before bed. Get off the computer! Take a bath. On the other hand, if you do wake up in the night, it is a very special time to meditate, especially around 4:00 A.M. (see the earlier suggestions on meditations for sleeplessness). I often get my most creative ideas in the middle of the night.

Nerve-wracking Situations

- *Crunched for time:* Deliberately schedule yourself to leave more time for everything. Even a few extra minutes between activities can make a significant difference; you can breathe and center yourself. Consider it part of creating healthy boundaries. Scheduling extra time helps to keep tension from accumulating in your nervous system (another tip for better sleep).

- *Driving:* Again, give yourself more time than you think you need so that you can minimize the panic and rush. If you're stuck in traffic, breathe and remember your sovereignty—don't give outside situations so much power over your well-being. Chant a mantra, get into your "Totem Animal," do the "Jazz Breath"—so what if other drivers laugh?

- *Waiting for someone:* Waiting is a wonderful chance to drop into meditative awareness. Rather than fret in impatience, use the time. Be with the sensuousness of your breath, do the "Simple Awareness" practice, catch up with yourself.
- *At the dentist:* Breathe slowly in your belly. Wiggle your toes to ground yourself in your feet. My hands tend to tense up at the dentist, so I hold my thumbs ("Thumbs Up") or massage my fingers. Think about how virtuous you will feel afterward!

STRETCH IT OUT

Animals always stretch before or after resting. Here are some easy stretches to do before or after meditation—or both! They can help wake you up in your body, bring more circulation, and relieve stiffness and discomfort. Let them be more like a gentle massage than a discipline, so don't force anything. Follow the pleasure principle: you want it to feel good!

AWAKENING TOUCH

Massage your arms, legs, hips, and thighs. Say hello to your belly and heart with your hands. Rub each finger long, massage into your palms and wrists. Give yourself love-taps all over your skin.

SHOULDER CIRCLES

Take a delicious deep breath and begin to circle your shoulders: forward, up toward your ears, around the back, and down. Do this eight times. Rest for a full breath, then reverse the direction. Circle back, up to your ears, forward and down, eight times. Think of this as lubrication for your bones.

REACH FOR IT

Reach your hands over your head and clasp them. Extend your arms and stretch up high. Exaggerate your breathing: inhale deeply through your nose, exhale through either your nose or mouth. Lean slightly into each side and feel the stretch from your waist all the way up through your arms. Feel your feet reaching down. Then relax and take a few breaths, noticing the increase of circulation. This can also be done lying down on your back.

LOLLYGAG HEAD ROLLS

Very gently let your chin sink down toward your chest, as if you were looking into your heart. Slowly let your head roll toward the right, your ear moving toward your shoulder. Go just to the side, not beyond it (don't roll your head back). Then roll forward again and do the same to the left. Feel the weight of your head and the release through your neck and shoulders. Repeat this rocking motion several times, as though you are being lulled in gentle waves. If you'd like to add the breath rhythm, inhale as you roll the head to the side, exhale as you release forward and down.

Spine Wave

In a sitting or standing position, slowly sway through your spine, gently curving forward and back, and side to side. Undulate softly and be aware of your entire spine. Let your head go with the movement, as though it is floating on top of the waves.

Wiggling Fingers and Toes

This can also be done lying down. Stretch your legs and arms out in any direction and move your feet and hands, as if to tickle the space with your fingers and toes. Wiggle each finger and toe, curl them all up, and spread them wide. Breathe fully.

Face and Jaw Release

Open your mouth and make the shape of the vowels—*ah, ay, ee, oo, uuu*. Say them silently, then whisper them, then let the sound come out strong. Feel the inside of your mouth, your teeth and tongue, how your lips move as you shape the sound. Bring your attention to the rest of your face. Open your eyes and look around, wriggle your nose and eyebrows. Go ahead and play, be silly, let go!

Scalp Massage

This is very relaxing—you'll love it! Starting at the top of your forehead, bring the first two fingers of both hands to your hairline, press firmly, and make little circles. Slowly move down, massaging along the hairline toward your ears. Pull the earlobes gently (this stimulates lots of meridians). Massage again in front of the ears, down your jaw, and all the way back up. Take a full minute to do this. Bring your hands to the top of your head and gently massage your scalp. See if you can feel the skin loosen and slide over your skull. Finally, flutter your fingers very lightly all over your face, like little butterfly kisses on your eyelids, cheeks, and lips.

Slinky Thing

If you don't have a carpet, use a couple of blankets on the floor for padding. Lie down in any position and take a minute to relax with your breath. Before you even begin to move, invite the sense of awakening lusciously, like some exotic creature in the jungle or a plant unfurling into the sun. Gradually let your body unfold—curling, rolling, and reaching with pleasure. Breathe, sigh, gurgle, groan. Rather than specific stretches, feel how natural and organic your movement can be. This is about luxuriating in flow with no particular demand. This is my favorite way to begin my dance yoga classes; it creates an atmosphere of ease and sensuality that really opens us up.

All Fours

We carry the wisdom of our four-legged friends within our own bodies. This stretch puts us in touch with our creaturehood and expands our sense of being human. Let it feel good, like a moving massage. Don't push. Each body has its range and limits, so always honor the feedback from yours.

On all fours, feel how your hands and knees meet the ground. If on a hard floor, use blankets or a pad to cushion your knees. Gently and slowly begin to curve your spine, arcing up, down, side to side. Now let your elbows bend lightly and move your shoulders so that your chest and head can sway slowly and fluidly. Feel how your belly and breasts dance over the earth. Breathe. Now get into your pelvis and notice how it tilts every which way. Imagine a tail extending out from your tailbone. What variety of tail do you have today? Long, sassy, full, and fluffy? Let it swish around and extend out behind you shamelessly. Now become more aware of your breath. Let your exhalation become audible and give yourself permission to make any sound that wants to come. Enjoy the freedom, sensuous power, and earthy connectedness of your movement.

When you tire or feel complete, you can gently sit back on your heels and curl down over your thighs, resting your arms. Or curl up on your side or simply lie on your back and relax into the ground for a couple of minutes.

SOFT EYES

The eyes are keys to the whole nervous system; they hold stress and any frozen trauma. Relaxing and softening them is a deep relief. If you work at a computer or read a lot, this is a good one for you. This is especially wonderful after the face and scalp massage.

Feel the little muscles all around the eye sockets, the skin of the eyelids, your brows. Wiggle your eyebrows slightly. Now notice your normal gaze. Even when the eyes are closed, they tend to stare in some direction. Gently release any fixity to your focus. Slowly let your gaze shift without moving your head, as though your eyes are just floating around in your head. Try this with your eyes both open and closed, looking slightly up, down, diagonally, side to side—everywhere in your field of vision.

Then, with closed eyes, gently bring your fingertips to touch the eyelids, the brows, the skin under and at the outer edges of the eyes. Let the soft touch help to relax them even more, then simply rest and enjoy the softness. Slowly open your eyes just a slit, then gradually a little more, staying soft. Let them effortlessly receive the light, color, and shapes around you. Take plenty of time to make a transition.

People sometimes think they are supposed to focus on their third eye when they meditate, so they glue their inner gaze to their forehead. Instead, always remember to let your eyes be soft and free to move.

❧ MEDITATIONS

Open Your Arms to Life

This is a wonderful meditation to do at the beginning of the day or before an important event. Sit comfortably for several moments to settle in and become present. When you are ready, stand with your feet hip-width apart in a powerful but open stance. Face toward the direction that feels most intense, for example, the heart of the city, or your lover's house. Take another minute or two to establish yourself there. Keep your eyes open so that you really see the outer world.

Bring your attention to your breath. Appreciate how its movement weaves you into the fabric of life—flowing inside and out, over and over again. Sense how it comes into your lungs, expanding through your chest and touching into your heart center.

When you are ready, let your arms float up into a wide embrace. Notice how in this position both the front and the back of your heart are open, streaming energy out through your arms and hands.

Now welcome every possible experience you will have today. Imagine everything—all the possible fun, the challenges, the difficult situations, the variety of personalities you will encounter, and what it may feel like to be with them. Think of how you want to be present to it all. Open your energy. Breathe with the quality and atmosphere you would like to create.

Breathe into your heart and continue to welcome all the energy. Accept your joy, your fear, your wonder, your excitement—and all the love that is in your heart. Percolate with your passion for life.

As a closing gesture, anchor these feelings into your body by bringing your hands to your heart. Close your eyes and take a breath or two. Then ease yourself out into action.

Let Your Sound Go Forth

After this meditation, be sure to take some time to bask in the aftereffects. Begin by sitting for several minutes to become present. Orient yourself to the space around you, eyes either open or closed.

Bring your hands to your belly and connect with the movement of your breath. Massage your abdomen, then draw your hands upward, massaging until they come to rest at your upper chest under the base of the throat. Gently tap that area a few times (awaken your thymus). Connect with the movement of your breath as you sense it there. Massage that entire area, around your neck and gently through your face and scalp. Relax your arms and let your hands rest wherever is comfortable. Moisten your lips, swallow a couple of times, move your mouth around.

Now gather your energy and sit so that your spine is soft but tall. Breathe fully and begin to imagine sending your essence out into the world. Where and how do you want to connect? What do you want to communicate? Stay with that awareness but bring your attention inward to sense the quality of energy that wants to move out. Now make your exhalation audible and listen to its sound for several breaths. Visualize energy flowing through the channel of your throat. What sound wants to come?

When you are ready, let your breath turn into vocal sound. Open your mouth. Let the sound emerge; take your time to explore until you find the sound that seems just right for you . . . *o, om, ah*—anything at all. Let it expand outward so that the space itself receives the impact of your vibration. Send it out clearly, boldly, lovingly. Let the vibration touch the whole world. Sing your sound to the stars.

᠔✸ GOING FURTHER

The Figure 8 Movement Meditation

This is a movement meditation on the rhythm of in-and-out, the free flow of creative energy between your inner world and the outer world.

After taking plenty of time to sink in, or after any other meditation, begin this movement gesture. Do this for five minutes, but don't expect to feel anything at first.

Begin with your hands resting, palms upward in your lap. Draw your fingertips in toward your lower belly and sweep them up the middle of your torso to your heart. As you move upward with your hands, you are saluting and activating the core energies of pelvis, belly, solar plexus, heart, and throat. When your hands approach your throat, begin to move them outward. Curve to flow down and out with your hands, as though giving a gift, until your arms are extended. Sweep upward and then begin to draw inward, cycling down to your belly and then up again through the heart.

Continue with the full cycle. Let the speed vary and, as your muscles get used to the movement, go as fast as you like. Then slow down gradually more and more, so that you smoothly and effortlessly glide through the dance.

If viewed from the side, this gesture would describe a figure 8, or two circles conjoined at one point (∞). This symbol is also used as the infinity sign. The motion does seem like an eternal gesture, the archetypal connection between your personal self and the universe.

Continue to explore the movement and contemplate the creative cycle of giving and receiving that it embodies. Embrace this movement as a ritual expression of your relationship to the infinite dance of life.

At Home in the Universe

This body scan is a meditation about the body in relationship to the universe. You can also use it at the end of another meditation to reorient and prepare to enter the world. Consider this: to be in a body, to be in your body, is not an experience of isolation, but an experience of relatedness.

Take a few moments to settle in, letting your senses catch up with you in the present moment. Then begin to scan through your body.

After resting your awareness in the area of your eyes for a few seconds, move your attention upward to your forehead and the top of your head. Then let it touch your lips, your jaws, your ears, the back of your head, your neck. Delicately sweep your awareness through each area, rest there for a few seconds, and move on.

Lovingly dwell in your breasts, your shoulders and arms, your spine behind the heart area. Slide down your back to your sacrum and tailbone, then wrap around to embrace your belly and pelvis. Dwell there for a few seconds. Then let your attention flow down your legs into your feet. Now encompass your entire body with your awareness.

Next, become aware of the space around your body. Place yourself inside the room, inside your house or apartment. Then become aware of your house in the midst of your neighborhood. Pay attention to the relationship of your body to your house in your city, then in your house in your city in its region, and then the continent. Feel your body in the house in the city in the region on the continent and then on all the continents. Extend your awareness to include each great landmass and body of water.

Now dwell in the ecstatic relationship of your body to the entire planet. When you get that sense, embrace your body in relationship to the sun, then the moon. Add the whole solar system, then the galaxy, then billions of galaxies. Now become aware of your body in relationship to the space within which the galaxies spin. Rest within the universal body, simply breathing.

Finally, begin to reverse the process, going from the cosmic to the individual. Bring your attention back through each stage of connection until you rest within your distinct self, your individual body.

Take a few minutes to imagine yourself moving in your daily world with this universal connection living inside you. Open your eyes very slowly, continuing to bridge your inner experience with the outer reality. When you're ready, go out and live it up!

&⁊ REFLECTIONS

- What have you discovered about your enthusiasm for life?
- Do you have a vision for yourself? For your community? For humanity?
- Cherish the life you have been given. What more wants to unfold?
- What friends and allies can support the life you want to live?
- What is one simple action you can take this week to move toward your dreams?

LATE-NIGHT MUSING

> ✒ My friend Carolyn Stevens, the late analyst and president of the C. G. Jung Institute of Chicago, had a pithy response to my query about the theories of masculine and feminine. "After all this time, I now just think that whatever women do *is* the feminine."

Our understanding of the cosmos changes as our consciousness evolves. Developments in scientific technology continually revolutionize our model of the universe, and as collective consciousness unfolds, we embrace surprising, sometimes shocking discoveries. We undergo paradigm shifts, which change forever how we perceive the world and our place within it.

A new cosmic vision of the feminine is emerging; it glimmers just beyond the veil of our awareness. Assumptions about "the feminine principle" have gone unquestioned, unexamined—unevolving—for millennia. Women have sought some reference beyond our cultural bias by looking to ancient archetypes of female wisdom. I certainly have, and those secrets are included in this book. They are empowering, indeed. But as valuable as they are, it occurs to me ever more strongly that the old forms are based on a much different world and stage of consciousness. As I ponder in the middle of the night, in the center of the darkness, I muse: What if something more, something newly female, is coming into being? What if it can only form through the engagement of women's attention—united feminine attention that until now has not been free?

After fifteen billion years, give or take a couple billion, consciousness has evolved within matter, and human beings can now participate in our own creation. It has taken all this time for us to conceive these questions, much less partake in the birth of something more. Perhaps our recent discovery of dark matter and the lessons it holds have something to do with it—who knows?

Meditation is a gentle midwife for the emergence of this new reality. As I listen in the silence and peer through the cosmic veil, I sense the shimmer of something nascent, something growing but as yet unseen. She is evolving as humanity evolves. Just as beings have incarnated at crucial points in human development (Moses, Buddha, Jesus), so too She is being born—not as an individual woman but as a knowing brought forth through us all. The entire globe is vibrating with change; the contractions have begun. What revelation is dawning now as women are awakening? What needed energy is coming into the world?

If you think this sounds radical, you are correct. It is a radical departure from the known, a radical plunge into the mystery within us all. It is up to women now to take on the quest, to share this vision that is ours to discover and unfold. We are at the frontier of consciousness; we are explorers, and it's exciting! Let's be surprised. Let's be shocked. How much freedom can we stand?

References and Recommendations

We suggest the following books as additional support for each chapter of *Secrets*. The right book at the right time can be a wonderful friend, a retreat, an advance, and food for the soul. It can speak to you more intimately than your best friend. Some of these have been best-sellers and are readily available; others were published by tiny presses and will have to be special-ordered. Thanks to computers and the Internet, your local bookstore can instantly locate almost any book ever published.

INTRODUCTION

Throughout the text we have, of course, changed the names of all the women who have shared their stories, to respect the privacy of their inner world.

The Feminine Face of God by Sherry Ruth Anderson and Patricia Hopkins (Bantam Doubleday Dell, 1992) is one of the first books to take on the problem of modern American women doing spiritual practices designed for the male celibates of Asia. They talked to many women meditators, and the book has great stories of women finding their own way. One message rings clearly through these stories: you can't imitate anyone else's spirituality. In the end, meditation is about coming home to rest in your own unique self, and much of what people do in the name of spirituality seems to lead them far, far away from themselves.

Carl G. Jung wrote extensively about the problems encountered by Westerners doing Asian meditative practices. His *Psychology and Religion: West and East* (Bollingen, 1969)—a huge academic tome that weighs three pounds—is a compilation of many different essays. The last two sections of the book are the most interesting for our purposes: they contain reprints of introductions that Jung was asked to write for the first editions of *The Tibetan Book of the Great Liberation,* the *I Ching,* and Suzuki's *Introduction to*

Zen Buddhism. His introductory essays are dense but full of penetrating insights. We have found that his criticism of Westerners trying to imitate the East rings true, year after year. Although he was writing in the early part of the twentieth century, his thinking is still way ahead of everyone else's. Order this book from a library some day and read the chapters "Yoga and the West" and "The Psychology of Eastern Meditation."

To understand how utterly simple meditation is, reading Herbert Benson is a real help. Benson, a cardiologist at Harvard Medical School, has been doing research on the physiology of meditation for more than thirty years and has published dozens of scientific studies and half a dozen books on the topic. He explains the medical benefits of meditation and gives bare-bones simple ways to practice. Benson has worked hard over the decades not to be a guru and not to mystify everything so as to dazzle the yokels. Read either *Timeless Healing: The Power and Biology of Belief* (with Marg Stark, Scribner, 1996) or *Beyond the Relaxation Response* (with William Proctor, Times Books, 1984).

Meditation Made Easy (HarperSanFrancisco, 1998) by Lorin Roche is a friendly step-by-step guide to meditating. It contains instructions for twenty or so meditation techniques, plus a procedure for adapting the techniques to fit your individual life. The book is designed to be read a bit at a time and then consulted when you encounter an experience you want to know how to handle—such as a great many thoughts, or sleepiness, or restlessness.

Healing Mind, Healthy Woman by Alice Domar and Henry Dreher (Delta, 1997) has a medical perspective on how a woman can use meditation to benefit her health and reviews some of the scientific literature on the health benefits of meditation.

For an approach to evolving your daily meditation practice that integrates sports, diet, martial arts, and special movement exercises, read *The Life We Are Given* by George Leonard and Michael Murphy (Putnam, 1995). Although they do not talk at all about the feminine, they are huge fans of Eastern teachings and have done magnificent work in adapting them to the needs of modern Westerners. These two are real veterans, and between them they have a vast amount of experience.

Maharishi Mahesh Yogi was one of the Indian gurus who popularized meditation in the West in the 1960s. When Lorin became a teacher of Transcendental Meditation, he attended many of Maharishi's talks. To read more about TM, check out *Maharishi Mahesh Yogi on the Bhagavad-Gita* (Arkana, 1990).

The information on the differences between male and female brains, and the inferences, comes from "The Sexual Brain" in *Mapping the Mind* by

Rita Carter (University of California Press, 1998, p. 71.) Many other sources confirm these conclusions.

His Holiness the Dalai Lama urges people to be happy in their own lives and not try to be monks. In June 1997, he gave talks in Los Angeles based on the Indian Buddhist classic, *The Precious Garland; an Epistle to a King,* by Acarya Nagarjuna, a monk who lived in the 2nd century. A special edition of that title (Wisdom Publications, 1997) was handed out to audience members. In Nagarjuna's text is a long, disgusting passage that desecrates the body, especially the female body, in a graphic admonition to kill out desire. Read this only if you want a blatant example of toxic attitudes to avoid. Fortunately, *The Art of Happiness: A Handbook for Living* by H.H. the Dalai Lama (Riverhead Books, 1998) has a much more inviting tone.

Psychoanalyst Wolfgang Lederer wrote a devastatingly honest book about misogyny, *The Fear of Women.* It is out of print, but another book, *The Fear of the Feminine* by Erich Neumann, another analyst, is available (Erich Neumann and Boris Matthews, Princeton University Press, 1994). Read this if you want to know more about men's hidden fear of women's power.

The Alice Walker quote, "At Home in Herself" on page xxxiv is from an interview with Sharon Salzberg (and Melvin McLeod) that appeared in *The Shambhala Sun* magazine, (January 1997). We thank them for their generous permission to quote. In one of the delights of the Internet, we e-mailed the *Sun* our request to quote, and received their permission less than twenty minutes later, even though their editor is in Canada and we are in California. Their archives, on the Web at www.shambhalasun.com, go back years and are a rich source of inspiration. For a subscription to *The Shambhala Sun,* write them at 1345 Spruce Street, Boulder, CO 80302-4886, or e-mail subscriptions@shambhalasun.com.

SECRET #1: CELEBRATE YOUR SENSES

"Every human being possesses an effective internal health maintenance system": Robert Ornstein and David Sobel, *Healthy Pleasures* (Addison-Wesley, 1989), p. 25. This book is unusual in that it presents important findings on brain science and yet is extremely readable, entertaining, and full of common sense. Two thumbs up for these two rascals. Ornstein and Sobel aren't just scientists; they are mystic-scientists, in our opinion. And because they have been working in the field for so long, they are not afraid to say: "Enjoy yourself. Take deep, sensuous pleasure in every aspect of your life—it'll be good for your health. Let your meditation be a healthy pleasure. We're scientists, so what we say must be true." In addition to their books, they publish the *Mind/Body Health Newsletter*.

Autobiography of a Yogi by Paramahansa Yogananda (Crystal Clarity Publications, 1994) is a poignant and entertaining story of Yogananda's encounters with many of the great teachers and saints of India. He describes the stages of his spiritual awakening, and the book has long been recognized as a classic.

A Natural History of the Senses by Diane Ackerman (Vintage Books, 1991) is a marvelous read. A poet, Ackerman revels in the physiology of the human sensory apparatus. At some point in life every human being on earth should read this book slowly and then go out into daily life and see it (and smell and taste and hear it) anew.

SECRET #2: HONOR YOUR INSTINCTS

"I'll literally excuse myself and sit on the toilet somewhere": Goldie Hawn shared these earthy jewels in interviews with *Health* (February 2000) and *Good Housekeeping* (July 1, 1997).

A different light is shed on the marvels of the instincts in each of the following books:

The Three Faces of Mind by Elaine de Beauport, with Aura Sofia Diaz (Quest Books, 1996) is a very clear exposition of the basic instincts and how they relate to areas of the brain. In particular, we love chapter 13, "Crossing the Threshold of the Unconscious into the Basic Brain," which is on the web at http://motley-focus.com/~timber/crossing.html.

The Gift of Fear by Gavin De Becker (Little, Brown and Co., 1997) is a unique book about learning to notice your intuition and self-protection instinct. De Becker is an expert on stalkers, and the book is full of stories of cases he has worked on. The central theme is how to read and act on the signals that tell you, "You are in danger." About half of everyone's meditation time seems to be taken up in what we call "signal processing," so if you get better at it, you may have fewer thoughts during meditation. De Becker makes a real contribution to understanding how to honor fear and thus reduce the amount of time you spend in pointless, unnecessary fear.

Why Zebras Don't Get Ulcers by Robert Sapolsky (W. H. Freeman and Co., 1998) is a great read for anyone interested in the physiology of stress—what happens in the body whenever we are startled, afraid, or angry, either for a moment or over a long period of time. Sapolsky is professor of biological sciences and neuroscience at Stanford University and a highly entertaining writer.

Deep Play by Diane Ackerman (Random House, 1999) is a romp through the literature on the human instinct for play—a much-neglected topic. This book is a good resource for those of us who are too serious in our approach to things and need help in developing a playful approach to meditation.

The Intuitive Body by Wendy Palmer (North Atlantic Books, 1994) may be hard to find. The publisher's address is P.O. Box 12327, Berkeley, CA 94712. This is one of the few books by a woman martial artist, and it is as much about meditation as it is about aikido, an exceptionally sublime martial art. She describes her experiences with the human energy field and the subtle bodily sensations that go with sensing other people's intentions. There is a great deal of wisdom here about how to move through the world and stay centered, and how to turn attacks into opportunities to wake up.

SECRET #3: CLAIM YOUR INNER AUTHORITY

In her *Anatomy of the Spirit: The Seven Stages of Power and Healing* (Harmony Books, 1996), Carolyn Myss, Ph.D., correlates the three systems of the Christian sacraments, the Jewish Kaballah, and the Hindu *chakras*.

"Your ego must be integrated and functional if you are to survive and cope": *Homecoming: Reclaiming and Championing Your Inner Child* by John Bradshaw (Bantam Doubleday Dell, 1992), p. 257.

The ancient and venerable Hindu tradition has a model of authority and of the teacher-student relationship (the scriptures say the Guru is "Greater than God") that is utterly foreign to Westerners. *Karma Cola: Marketing the Mystic East* by Gita Mehta (Random House, 1990) is hilarious and required reading for anyone interested in Eastern meditation practices.

For a fresh take on the chakras, we recommend *Eastern Body, Western Mind: Psychology and the Chakra Sysem As a Path to the Self* (Ten Speed Press, 1996) and *Wheels of Life: A User's Guide to the Chakra System* (Llewellyn's New Age Series, 1987), both by Anodea Judith. Her work is an intelligent integration of psychology, metaphysics, and somatic therapy.

In *Truth or Dare* (HarperSanFrancisco, 1987) Starhawk talks about the difference between power-from-within and power-over. She has a unique, mystical voice in talking about women's issues. Starhawk is a witch—a good witch—and gives voice to a pagan, earth-embracing religion in which spirituality comes up from the ground, through your feet, and into your body.

Women of Wisdom by Tsultrim Allione (Routledge & Kegan Paul, 1984) brings to light the little-known lineage of women in Tibetan Buddhism, from the perspective of a contemporary American woman in that tradition.

For a long read with many, many good chapters, take a look at *The New American Spirituality* by Elizabeth Lesser (Random House, 1999). Lesser was one of the founders of the Omega Institute, a seminar center in New York that for many years has sponsored workshops on drumming, dancing, meditation, massage, and every other kind of so-called New Age training. In particular, read the section "Feminine Spirituality in a Masculine World."

SECRET #4: BE TENDER WITH YOURSELF

A Woman's Worth by Marianne Williamson (Random House, 1993) is a good short read about how not to be mean to yourself.

Barbara DeAngelis has been meditating devotedly since 1970 and writes knowingly on spiritual ideas from inside the female experience. *Secrets About Life Every Woman Should Know* (Hyperion, 1999) is a good place to start. DeAngelis knows how to combine an intense meditation practice with an equally intense "love life and a go-for-it attitude" toward the outer world.

Revolution from Within: A Book of Self-Esteem by Gloria Steinem (Little, Brown and Co., 1992) is a comprehensive tour of inner work from this well-known feminist and political activist. Ms. Steinem articulates the collective shame that many women carry and offers some ways to counter it.

Continuum is an elegant approach to healing movement developed by founder Emilie Conrad and Susan Harper. For information on workshops in your area, call their office (310) 453–4402 or visit their Web site: www.ContinuumMovement.com

SECRET #5: DWELL IN YOUR INNER SANCTUARY

The theory of the "tend and befriend" nature of women's response to stress has been researched by a team led by Dr. Shelley E. Taylor, professor of psychology at UCLA. Their report will be published in *Psychological Review*.

Women's Bodies, Women's Wisdom by Dr. Christiane Northrup (Bantam Doubleday Dell, 1998) is a comprehensive overview of women's health issues. Northrup marries conventional medicine with alternative medicine in a way that reveals their deep complementarity. She also puts out a newsletter, *Health Wisdom for Women,* that we eagerly read every month.

There are many goddesses, each with her own feeling tone. If you are interested in the Greek goddess archetypes, check out *The Moon and the Virgin: Reflections on the Archetypal Feminine,* by Nor Hall (New York: Harper & Row, 1980), *Pagan Meditations,* by Ginette Paris (Spring Publications, 1991), and *Goddesses in Every Woman,* by Jean Shinoda Bolen (Harper & Row, 1984). *Tantric Yoga and the Wisdom Goddesses* by David Frawley (Passage Press, 1994) gives an overview of the goddesses according to Hindu and Vedic knowledge. He also describes the chakras in the human body and their corresponding mantras and visualizations. This book may be hard to find; the publisher's address is P.O. Box 21713, Salt Lake City, UT, 84121.

SECRET #6: ANSWER THE CALL

We recommend *The Pregnant Virgin: A Process of Psychological Transformation* by Marion Woodman (Inner City Books, 1985). Woodman is a Jungian analyst and former English teacher. She writes with passion and poetry about the challenges involved in hearing, and answering, our inner calls.

Queen Maeve and Her Lovers: A Celtic Archetype of Ecstasy, Addiction, and Healing is by another Jungian psychoanalyst, Sylvia Perera (Carrowmore Books, 1999). Perera's writing is infused with the real-life experience of her clients and informed by fairy tales and myths. This tome is comprehensive and illuminating.

In *The Heroine's Journey* (Shambhala, 1990) Maureen Murdock discusses the many different ways in which a woman can be called to the adventure of exploring her feminine self. Drawing on Joseph Campbell's *The Hero with a Thousand Faces* (Bollingen Press, 1973), the book presents the hero's story from the female point of view and is full of feminine insight.

SECRET #7: RIDE YOUR RHYTHMS

"The impetuous seed of creation does not exactly come forth on little cat feet": Georgianne Cowan, "The Sacred Womb" in *The Soul of Nature: Visions of a Living Earth,* edited by Michael Tobias and Georgianne Cowan (Continuum Publishing Co., 1994), p. 189. This quote is used with the author's gracious permission.

A Woman's Book of Life: The Biology, Psychology, and Spirituality of the Feminine Life Cycle by Joan Boryshenko (Riverhead Books, 1998) discusses the spiritual phases of a woman's life in terms of biology. Boryshenko is one of the few Ph.D.s in anatomy who writes about meditation. This is an excellent book; we give it an A-plus.

Menopausal Years: The Wise Woman Way by Susun Weed (Ash Tree Publishing, 1992) offers "alternative approaches for women 30 to 90." Weed is an herbalist (of course, with a name like that), and she gives very helpful advice on many levels about the menopausal transition. I keep the book in my nightstand and refer to it often.

Coming into Our Own: Understanding the Adult Metamorphosis by Mark Gerzon (Delacorte Press, 1992) addresses the challenges and possibilities of midlife.

Maps to Ecstasy: A Healing Journey for the Untamed Spirit by Gabrielle Roth (New World Library, 1998) maps out a way of relating meditation and dance. For many women, dancing before meditation is an important and joyous warm-up that enriches the whole experience. Then meditation itself feels like a subtle internal dance.

Several years ago I attended a workshop with Angeles Arrien at Earth Trust in Malibu. She spoke there about seeing the four phases of life in some people's faces, and it stayed with me. There are no published sources of that information, but she has written a number of wise and helpful books.

The estimates for the number of people killed as heretics during the Inquisition come from *The Great Cosmic Mother: Rediscovering the Religion of the Earth* by Monica Sjöö and Barbara Mor (Harper & Row, 1987), p. 298. This scholarly work is filled with pithy facts, all of which are diligently referenced.

SECRET #8: SAY YES TO EVERY PART OF YOURSELF

Your Many Faces by Virginia Satir (Celestial Arts, 1978) is slightly more than one hundred pages long and exceptionally readable. Satir was widely regarded as a genius at therapy, and in *Your Many Faces* she maps out how to work with your inner subpersonalities or alter egos.

Core Transformation by Connirae Andreas, with Tamara Andreas (Real People Press, 1994), is a challenging read but worth it. Andreas's description of how to relate your inner selves to each other is unparalleled in clarity. In explaining how to turn your inner critics into inner allies, no one says it better. Another good book of hers is *Heart of the Mind* (Real People Press, 1989), which she wrote with her husband, Steve Andreas. This book clues you in on how your brain invents techniques as needed, all the time, to help you through your daily personal crises.

Motherpeace: A Way to the Goddess Through Myth, Art, and Tarot by Vicki Noble (HarperSanFrancisco, 1994) imparts a wealth of information about feminine archetypes and working with your inner parts. Consider exploring it just for the symbolism; it can be an incredible visual tool for accepting your inner characters and voices. A tarot deck, the *Motherpeace Tarot Deck* (United States Games Systems, 1993), goes with the book. In conception the book and deck are neo-Jungian and neo-pagan, so be ready for that angle of the mysteries if you approach this wonderful work.

The Dark Side of the Light Chasers by Debbie Ford (Penguin Putnam, 1998) is an excellent guide to working with your "dark side," the part of yourself you think is not spiritual and that you may feel you have to disown. The book is very readable and entertaining.

SECRET #9: REST IN SIMPLICITY

Simple Abundance by Sarah Ban Breathnach (Warner Books, 1995) is a delightful daybook to work with (a page a day for a year). We enjoy her tremendously. She does a beautiful job of talking about setting up your day so that meditation can fit into it and making your everyday world a home for your authentic, soulful self.

Gift from the Sea by Anne Morrow Lindbergh (Vintage Books, 1991) is a tiny book that is perfect to take to the beach or the riverbank or the grass in the backyard when you want to have a peaceful moment.

SECRET #10: DO NOT FEAR THE DEPTHS

The name for the "Descent to the Goddess" active imagination on page 222 comes from the groundbreaking work of that name by Sylvia Perera. *Descent to the Goddess: A Way of Initiation for Women* (Inner City Books, 1989) reveals the feminine mystery of descent through the Sumerian myth of Innanna and Ereshkigal.

Other precious resources for excavating your depths include:

Women Who Run with the Wolves by Clarissa Pinkola Estes (Ballantine, 1992) is a book by a skilled storyteller and Jungian analyst who recounts the feminine experience with poignancy and depth.

Knowing Woman: A Feminine Psychology by Lucy Claremont de Castillejo (Harper Colophon Books, 1974) and *The Way of All Women* by M. Esther Harding (Harper Colophon, 1975) are classics.

Woman, Earth, and Spirit: The Feminine in Symbol and Myth by Helen M. Luke (Crossroad Publishing Co., 1990) is a wonderful book that may be hard to find; the publisher's address is: 370 Lexington Ave., New York, NY 10017. Luke writes with a truly authentic voice about women's mysteries.

Women and Nature: The Roaring Inside Her by Susan Griffin (Harper Colophon Books, 1978) was one of the first books to challenge patriarchal assumptions and reconnect women to our natural source.

Care of the Soul by Thomas Moore (HarperCollins, 1992) is another great source of support.

SECRET #11: LOVE YOUR BODY

"Most women have lost that sense of power from their sexuality": Murdock, *The Heroine's Journey*, p. 114.

"As a woman returns from the descent, she reclaims her body": Ibid., p. 117.

"The Place Where You Are Right Now" is in *The Subject Tonight Is Love: Sixty Wild and Sweet Poems by Hafiz,* versions by Daniel Ladinsky (Pumpkin House Press, 1996).

Addiction to Perfection by Marion Woodman (Inner City Books, 1988) is about eating disorders but goes beyond that into the factors that lead a woman to cut herself off from her body. Lorin says that Woodman is one of the few people who write from deep inside the body, from the bone marrow where red blood cells are created; her words pulse with the human heartbeat.

Woman: An Intimate Geography by Natalie Angier (Houghton Mifflin, 1999) is a very sassy scientific exposé on recent findings in female biology.

Women's Intuition: Unlocking the Wisdom of the Body by Paula M. Reeves (Conari Press, 1999) is a guide to reclaiming your intuition through spontaneous movement. She explores at length one of our favorite topics—the way the body generates its own healing movements if we only give it a chance.

Women's Comfort Book by Jennifer Louden (HarperSanFrancisco, 1992), a guide to nurturing yourself, is laid out like a cookbook—very practical and recipe-oriented.

The Vagina Monologues by Eve Ensler (Villard, 1998) is the book based on the extraordinary performance of the same name. Ensler asked women to talk about their relationship to their vulvas and wombs, and the result is funny, moving, and profound.

In *The Soul of Sex* (HarperCollins, 1998), Thomas Moore, a monk for twelve years who became a therapist, writes about sex with humor, wonder, and reverence. He speaks about symptoms as symbols, and how to listen to their poetry, in his *Care of the Soul* (HarperCollins, 1992), p.161.

The Art of Sexual Magic by Margo Anand (Putnam, 1995) does a wonderful job of exploring the meditative and spiritual side of sexuality. This book glows with the love Anand put into it and contains a whole series of body explorations and meditations you can do to overcome your shame and embarrassment about your sexuality as you embrace it as an intrinsic part of your spiritual nature.

SECRET #12: LIVE IT UP

"You know what are hearts for?": Sharon Salzberg and Melvin McLeod, interview with Alice Walker, *Shambhala Sun* (January 1997).

The Artist's Way by Julia Cameron (J. P. Tarcher, 1992) is a savvy guide to recovering your creativity. It's the kind of book that, once you have read it, you love to just pick it up and read a paragraph or a page. We also recommend her later book, *The Vein of Gold* (Putnam, 1997). Both these books use meditation as a tool to get at what is deep inside you, to nurture it, and to bring it out into the world.

The Princessa: Machiavelli for Women by Harriet Rubin (Dell, 1998) is a lively guide to overcoming obstacles to thriving in the outer world. Rubin talks about wielding power in a female way and creating win-win situations. As Jesus exhorted us, we must be "wise as serpents, innocent as doves." Every meditator has to learn to use power well, or your meditation time will be filled with endless reviews of how you are *not* using power well.

Echo's Subtle Body: Contributions to an Archetypal Psychology by Patricia Berry (Spring Publications, 1982) provides many refreshing perceptions on the inner life and the constructs we use to describe it. Her essay, "The Dogma of Gender," examines the pitfalls of gender identity. She invites us to venture beyond the reductionist language of "masculine" and "feminine" into a deeper exploration of individuality. Pat's insights into dream, fantasy, and desire have shaped the field of archetypal psychology, and we hope to see more of her views in print.

James Hillman's work is a startling revisioning of the fundamentals of psychology. We recommend all of his writings. In *The Soul's Code: In Search of Character and Calling* (Warner Books, 1997), he proposes that each life is formed by an innate image, a creative daimon that calls that life to its destiny.

&

It could take easily ten or twenty years to work your way through this list—but then, we hope you will be meditating for at least that long. Always remember when reading to savor the words consciously. The truth about meditation is not "out there" in books or other people; it is "in here." When you read, the associations you make are important; the things you have forgotten and need to be reminded of are often the most useful. Your disagreements with the author, or realizations that you do not fit into the generalities he or she uses, provide the most useful, if uncomfortable, information. When you become uncomfortable in that special way, you can see where your individuality diverges from the generic, and from the herd.

Find poetry that moves your heart. Poetry speaks directly from and to the soul and can be a wonderful sharing of what cannot be said in ordinary language. We especially recommend the ancient poets Rumi, Kabir, and Hafiz. My favorite ancient poet, Mirabai, is one of the few female ecstatics whose works are in print.

Music Recommendations

Musical tastes are intensely individual, particularly in what creates a feeling tone helpful for meditation. That being said, here are some unusual pieces enjoyed by the women with whom we have worked.

SOFT AND GENTLE

Sunyata and *Offerings* by Vas

A BoneCroneDrone and *Weaving My Ancestors' Voices* by Sheila Chandra

Eight String Religion by David Darling

Himalaya, Yatra, and *Dorje Ling* by David Parsons

Shamanic Dream by Anugama

El Hadra: The Mystik Dance by Klaus Wiese et al.

Sustaining Cylinders, Ancient Leaves and *Planetary Unfolding* by Michael
    Stearns (Anything by him is wonderful)

The Lama's Chant by Lama Gyurmé and Jean-Philippe Rykiel

EMOTIONALLY EVOCATIVE

The Mirror Pool by Lisa Gerrard

Earth Heart by Vicki Hansen

Symphony #3 by Henryk Gorecki

Bach's cello solos

Gabriel Faure's *Requiem*

Passion: Music for "The Last Temptation Of Christ" by Peter Gabriel

Chronos and *Baraka* by Michael Stearns

Mass by Charles Bernstein

DRUM RHYTHMS

Percussive Environments by Jim McGrath

Medicine Trance by Professor Trance

At the Edge by Mickey Hart

About the Authors

CAMILLE MAURINE is a dancer who started meditating in 1972, and in 1975 began teaching meditation and body awareness in the context of her dance classes. Her training in healing includes twelve years as a practitioner of Essential Integration body therapy (1977–1989) and Continuum movement meditation since 1983. She has been involved with Transcendental Meditation, esoteric yoga, Zen, and Tibetan Buddhism, and has studied Jungian depth psychology. Over the years Camille has developed her own approach to inner work and creativity that integrates meditation, yoga, dance, and theater.

Camille creates one-woman shows and travels widely to give performances and workshops. She is creating a new work, "*Secrets*," as a performance adjunct to this book. Lorin and Camille also love traveling together to teach.

☙

LORIN ROCHE started meditating in 1968 in a research project on the physiology of meditation. Trained in 1970 as a meditation teacher, he has been active ever since, working with students from all walks of life. In 1975 he threw out the idea of importing meditation techniques from India and imposing them on Westerners and reinvented meditation from the ground up. He attended graduate school in social science at the University of California at Irvine. His master's thesis (1985) focused on the hazards of meditation and the crisis points in a meditator's development. He received his Ph.D. in 1987 for his study of the language that meditators use to describe their inner experiences. Lorin is grounded in the Himalayan meditation traditions, which he loves, but feels that women probably invented meditation. He is the author of *Meditation Made Easy*, also published by HarperSanFrancisco.

Acknowledgments

Ideas are always birthed out of a larger matrix of exploration. We would like to express our appreciation for some of the people who have been a significant influence along the way.

I, Camille, would like to acknowledge my friend Federico Montoya and his profound teachings on Essential Movement, which he shared with me in the late 1970s. I will be forever grateful to June Kounin, elder extraordinaire, for modeling the feminine strength that allowed me to delve to the bedrock of my soul—and that informs me still. I applaud my cherished ally and friend Emilie Conrad for the courage of her vision, for creating Continuum, and for articulating a radical understanding of the intelligence of the body. Thank you for your lively encouragement and our ongoing creative dialogues.

Special mention goes to the Jungian Women's Gathering—a group of wise and wooly analysts and a couple of extras such as myself—who met for ten years each June in Taos to plunge into our feminine depths. Your wisdom walks always with me in my bones. Deep gratitude to Medora Woods for her many levels of support, including a generous grant that permitted me to devote a year to writing. To my magnificent movement cohorts Susan Harper, Georgianne Cowan, and Stephanie Franz Rivera, deep appreciation for our circle of four, dancing with each other through a decade of life passages—births, deaths, divorces, and marriages.

Loving thanks to all my bosom buddies around the world, especially Louisa Putnam, Deanne Newman, Jessica Fleming, Katharine Lee, and Carol Zeitz, for keeping me company on the journey and tending the web of connectedness.

Lorin would like to thank Beulah Smith, his first meditation teacher. He is particularly grateful to his sister, Dale Lewis, for a lifetime of conversation. Drawing upon her experience with meditation, mothering, Co-Counseling, and teaching, Dale has made many perceptive contributions to this book. He'd also like to acknowledge the hundreds of women who over the last thirty-three years have shared their stories in such rich detail with him and who, by sharing, taught him to listen.

Much appreciation flows to our beloved agent, Gareth Esersky at the Carol Mann Agency in New York, for inventing such a friendly way of doing business. Many blessings to our editor Doug Abrams at HarperSanFrancisco for his insightful guidance, and to his assistant Renée Sedliar—thanks to you both for such enjoyable exchanges throughout production. Gratitude unbounded to our pal Ilene Segalove, who perseveringly supported, read, and honed the book with her unique and sassy take on things. Many thanks to our readers John Chamberlain, with his science and English teacher's eye, and Sara Staehle Urso, for sharing valuable comments.

I owe my commitment to passion, pleasure, and inner peace to my mother, Beverly Angelina (1926–71). A wildwoman before her time, she embodied the tragedy of trapped female energy, illuminating the struggle through her life and death in Technicolor so that I could clearly get the point and transmute the legacy.

I would also like to state the obvious: timeless appreciation of my husband, Lorin, for being such a spirited warrior on behalf of women and for standing with me in these creative fires. Thank you for your hearty laugh, for teasing me when I'm too serious, and for the joyous miracle we live.

How to Reach Us

For information on lectures, workshops, videos and tapes, performances, and other writings, come visit our web sites: www.camillemaurine .com and www.lorinroche.com. If you have questions, comments, or experiences you would like to share, please e-mail us at: secrets@camillemaurine .com.

You can also contact us through our publisher:
HarperSanFrancisco
353 Sacramento Street
Suite 500
San Francisco, CA 94111-3653
(415) 477-4400